THE REJUVENATION SOLUTION

Age in Reverse—7 Proven Medical Breakthroughs That Prevent Disease and Make You Feel Years Younger

Robert D. Willix, Jr., MD

Health Communications, Inc.
Deerfield Beach, Florida

www.hcibooks.com

This book is not intended as a substitute for the advice/medical care of the reader's physician, nor is it meant to dissuade or discourage the reader from the advice of his or her physician. The reader should regularly consult with a physician in matters relating to his or her health, and especially with regard to symptoms that may require a diagnosis. Any eating or lifestyle regimen should be undertaken under the direct supervision of the reader's physician.

Library of Congress Cataloging-in-Publication Data
is available through the Library of Congress

© 2019 Robert D. Willix, Jr., MD

ISBN-13: 978-07573-2287-7 (Paperback)
ISBN-10: 07573-2287-5 (Paperback)
ISBN-13: 978-07573-2289-1 (ePub)
ISBN-10: 07573-2289-1 (ePub)

All rights reserved. Printed in the United States of America. No part of this publication may be reproduced, stored in a retrieval system, or transmitted in any form or by any means, electronic, mechanical, photocopying, recording, or otherwise, without the written permission of the publisher.

HCI, its logos, and marks are trademarks of Health Communications, Inc.

Publisher: Health Communications, Inc.
    3201 S.W. 15th Street
    Deerfield Beach, FL 33442–8190

Cover photo design and illustrations by Larissa Hise Henoch
Interior design and formatting by Lawna Patterson Oldfield

I would like to dedicate this book to all of my
many teachers and mentors. These are the men that never
gave up on me and my dreams. They molded me into a
doctor, author, teacher, and a spiritual man.

Tony Verducci and Pete Calgagno, the high school
football coaches that kept me off of the streets and taught me
life lessons that continue to serve me today.

My mentors, Herbert Sloan, MD, C. Gardner Child, MD,
and Marvin Kirsch, MD, who never ceased instructing me to
become the best surgeon I could be.

George Sheehan, MD, a philosopher, cardiologist,
and pioneer of sports medicine and one of my best friends
who ignited in me the spark that allowed me to leave
cardiovascular surgery. George saw the path to healing and proved
to me that surgery is a lesser weapon than exercise.

The Q'ero shaman of Peru for their endless dedication to a
healing lineage that will be lost if we do not stop and listen to the
ancients. A very special tribute to Don Manuel Quispe,
Jose Luis Hererra, and Alberto Villoldo.

CONTENTS

INTRODUCTION

Everyone wants to stay young, which is why everyone is still searching for the Fountain of Youth.

Well, search no more. In *The Rejuvenation Solution,* I reveal how to slow the aging process and prevent the diseases of aging. Based on meticulously researched clinical evidence, in addition to my forty-plus years of working with thousands of patients, this book provides an account of breakthrough anti-aging treatments that stop you from feeling and looking old.

Let me be upfront with you right now: *There is a secret to slowing down aging.* This secret is that you can't rely on just one particular treatment or approach, as other anti-aging experts contend, but rather on an interrelated series of anti-aging game changers. By harnessing all of them, you can improve the quality and duration of your life span and maintain superb health and youthfulness all through life. Until now, no one has talked about them *collectively* as the true secret to slowing the aging process.

But the tide is turning. Even some of the most conservative scientists now believe that the human life span has the potential of 122 years. Then, of course, there is the issue of "health span"—the number of years in which you live as healthy and productively as possible. It would be amazing to live 122 years and have a health span of 122 years, wouldn't it?

Most of us get concerned about aging and would love to live that long and remain healthy and vigorous that long. Of course, aging is something that is extremely visible. You can see it happening to yourself and to others. What's making it happen? And is there anything that can be done to regulate it?

I've spent my career and my life answering these questions and pursuing scientific methods to slow biological aging and increase life span and health span in humans—something medical authorities say can't be done, even though most people want to see aging and the diseases of aging vanquished.

One thing you should know: I am not your conventional physician. I draw from a broad range of philosophies and alternative approaches to improve a person's well-being and state of health. I have journeyed to the sacred mountains of Peru and sat with the descendants of the Inca traditional healers, the Q'ero Shamans. I have observed how Ayurvedic doctors use the pulse to feel the energy of the physical imbalances that cause symptoms. I learned from a qigong master to observe energy flowing from his hands and how to harness that energy to heal.

I prefer to treat diseases and conditions with herbs, nutritional supplements, and bioidentical hormones over prescription drugs. I believe wholeheartedly in stress management techniques to deal with anxiety and depression over anti-depressants and anti-anxiety drugs. And, I typically "prescribe" exercise as a form of healing.

One patient came to me years ago with chronic obstructive pulmonary disease (COPD), usually a condition that gets worse over time. He was a former principal of a school in San Francisco, California, but had to quit his job at the young age of fifty-six because he could no longer carry out activities of daily living. The first thing I wanted him to do was work out. He objected, believing that exercise could not change his life.

I convinced him to give it a try—with both aerobic exercise and weight training. He stuck with it. By the end of one year, he was walking four miles a day on the treadmill and had returned to a normal lifestyle. Four years later, he was still at it, even walking the hills of San Francisco with his grandkids. And the COPD? It was cured with exercise.

I consider myself as a healer, although I was conventionally trained as a heart surgeon. In fact, I have undergone the rites to become an Altomesayoq shaman in the Q'ero tradition, understood to be the "energy weavers," responsible for originating the spiritual and nature-based life philosophy. And I have been given the Quechua (South American) name *Huamani* (pronounced *Waa Ma Knee*), which means "Hawk Spirit."

Let's Pick It Up

I started searching for these answers at a very young age. When I was thirteen years old, I witnessed the senseless deaths of my two best friends—tragedies that would alter my life forever.

Louie, a buddy since grade school, was found dead in an alley from a heroin overdose. The needle was still in his arm. It wasn't suicide; I knew him well enough to know he would never take his own life.

The other friend, nicknamed "Crazy Benny," was stabbed to death after attempting to quit a gang called the Roman Juniors.

Both deaths left an imprint on me that life was very fragile, and I didn't want to die young.

I wanted desperately to escape my low-income, gang-ridden neighborhood as quickly as I could. It was about as tough a place as they come. And they come pretty tough in Newark, New Jersey, where I was born and raised by an Irish father and an Italian mother. Every morning, I'd wake up, thank God for a new day, pray, and meditate. Even now, I start my day in the same way.

I became interested in meditation after reading a book called *The Return of Rishi* by Deepak Chopra, MD. It focuses on a technique called primordial sound meditation, referring to the sound that occurred in the universe at the time and place of your birth.

To find out more about this, I called Dr. Chopra. He politely asked me if I already practiced daily meditation to which I answered, "No." He advised me to learn transcendental meditation (TM) and practice it for two years prior to learning my primordial sound. I found a TM teacher who asked me to meditate twenty minutes twice a day for one consecutive year. I followed the directions faithfully. Since 1987, I have been meditating, using TM, for twenty minutes twice a day. I believe that it is one of the most powerful practices, along with exercise and nutrition, in prolonging my productive life.

I spent the majority of my youth playing sports, and I loved it. From age three on, I went to baseball games with my dad who was a very good amateur baseball player. As I got a little older, I joined a little league baseball team. Where I lived, there was pressure and temptation to join a gang, but thankfully, athletics helped me stay out of trouble.

Moved in part by Benny's death, I asked my father to train me to be ready to play high school football. My reasoning was that if I could get a football scholarship to college, this would be my ticket out of the neighborhood. I also wanted to be the first kid in my neighborhood and the first in a very large Italian family (my mother was the youngest of thirteen children) to go to college.

My dad had been a very good football player in high school. Too poor to attend college, he went to work for Prudential Insurance as soon as he graduated. Dad kept the same job until he retired at sixty-four years of age.

"Being a good football player will be tough," he replied. "But if you're willing to work hard, I can help you."

And so began my training.

We spent our summers in a little cottage in South Belmar, New Jersey. Every morning at 5 AM, before taking the one-hour train ride to Newark,

Dad would get up, take me to the beach, and run me through a routine. The calisthenics and drills were so grueling and the mornings so hot that I began to question my decision after the first week. I knew my father would not let me down, however, and I did not want to disappoint him by admitting I wanted to quit. He was making a huge sacrifice for me by getting up that early and working with me.

At the conclusion of every practice, he would make me run forty-yard dashes hard in the soft sand. At the time, I remember thinking that my dad, at age thirty-eight, was very old yet quite athletic. After the last sprint, he'd say, "Let's pick it up," and he would race me to the finish line. I could never beat him, not even by my senior year in high school.

As for my goal of playing football? My dad's training and belief in me paid off. I became the first freshman in the history of Seton Hall Prep to become the starting fullback.

My dad did an incredible job instilling in me that pursuit for maximum effort. He helped me get in tune with my body, striving for excellence, and learning that we're so much more resilient than we give ourselves credit for being.

Many years later, after I had become a hot-shot heart surgeon, I was visiting my parents at that same small cottage in South Belmar. At 5:00 one morning, I was sneaking out of the house to go on a run when I felt a tap on my shoulder.

"Where are you going?" asked my dad.

"I'm off on a five-mile run."

"Me too!"

I tried to talk him out of it—after all, I was thirty-four, and he was sixty. I did not want to go running with this old man! Needless to say, I could not shake him. He was determined. I was sure that I'd drop him at some point.

We jogged up to the boardwalk, which was located at the same beach where he had trained me to play football, and started to run. After four miles, he looked at me and uttered those infamous words, "Hey, Bobby, let's pick it up."

I knew a man of sixty could not beat me. There was no way. On that last mile, we ran stride for stride until the last 100 yards or so, and then what did I see? That old familiar sight: Dad's backside pulling in front of me. I was left wondering, "Will he ever get old?"

The next year, I invited my dad and mom to go to Hawaii, where I was going to run my first marathon, the famous Honolulu Marathon. I was shocked when Dad said, "I would like to run it with you."

"No, Dad, the marathon is 26.2 miles."

"I know the distance. I finished the New York City Marathon this year."

I was dumbfounded. My father was sixty-one years old!

Fast forward to mile twenty-four in that marathon: Stride for stride until we had only 2.2 miles to go, Dad said, "Hey, Bobby, let's pick it up."

I took one look at him and said, panting, "I'm sorry, I have nothing left in the tank. You go ahead!" And he did, beating me by more than eight minutes in the last two miles and 365 yards of the marathon.

At that marathon, I realized that I wanted to know more about how humans age because I wanted to age the way my dad did—which was hardly aging at all! What could I learn about aging from my dad and others, like my friend George Sheehan, MD, Jack LaLanne, and Norman Shealy, MD? What causes aging? Can you slow the process down? What can be done to reverse the effects of aging? Finding the answers to those questions became my life's work.

Dad went on to win medals in the senior Olympics for running, cycling, javelin, and shot put—all won after he turned seventy-five. He died while training for a London Marathon in his mid-eighties. No cause of death was ever detected.

I never forgot his mantra: Let's pick it up. He was a role model to me for aging well—or rather, aging slowly. He showed me that aging doesn't have to be that hard, and that we can all slow the rate at which we will age. This starts with *picking it up*—enhancing and accelerating—the cellular processes that cause the body to gradually decline with age. These cellular processes are affected by nutrition, lifestyle, exercise, stress, and other influences within our control. By picking up even small amounts of healthful behavior, we can delay these processes and age much more slowly.

I've always realized that the time we have on earth is very short, and I feel that we must strive to be the best at all levels of physical and mental accomplishment. Stay healthy. Laugh a lot. Love your life and the people in it. In other words, *pick it up*—and you'll stay young longer.

From Heart Surgery to Integrative/Anti-Aging Medicine

My dad and his active lifestyle were the initial catalysts for my subsequent journey toward what would become my destiny and destination—anti-aging medicine. But there were other sparks along the way as I began and pursued my medical career.

I studied for my MD/PhD at the University of Missouri Medical School where I graduated eighth in my class. During this time, I fell in love with surgery. I never completed my PhD but did attend the prestigious University of Michigan for my straight surgical internship and general and cardiac surgery training.

As a resident, I was invited to attend a medical conference in 1973 where health guru Nathan Pritikin was speaking about nutrition—and how his low-fat diet, based on vegetables, fruits, and grains, could not only promote weight loss but also prevent and control many of the world's leading killers, including diabetes, hypertension, and heart disease.

The doctors in the audience booed him off the stage. After all, he wasn't a doctor. What did he know? Nathan was an engineer; how could he tell these brilliant physicians the cause of disease?

I, on the other hand, had a "God experience." What if this guy is right? I wanted to know more. My natural curiosity and love of research sent me on a quest to learn more about the link between proper nutrition and health. The knowledge I uncovered was so compelling that I eventually became a vegetarian in 1977. Prior to my "conversion," I was chowing down on twelve-ounce steaks every night for dinner, straight from the seventy-acre farm I lived on, and my freezer was full of animal meat. But after I made the switch to vegetarianism, I experienced an amazing side effect: I felt rejuvenated and many years younger.

I learned how critical other lifestyle factors were, too. I was working more than one hundred hours a week and smoking a half a pack of cigarettes a day. And exercise? My only form of physical activity was picking up a scalpel. I was on track to becoming another medical statistic, and that frightened me. So I quit smoking in 1975. I began a stress management program, and I resumed running. Every single bad habit I changed helped me feel better and better—and naturally younger.

I didn't know it at the time because I was so busy becoming a successful heart surgeon, but I was developing what would later become significant tenets of my anti-aging program.

I was ultimately drawn to the surgical program at the University of South Dakota and became the first board-certified heart surgeon in the state. I went on to start the first open-heart surgery program in South Dakota.

It took years to train my team in South Dakota to perform open-heart surgery. We trained in the animal lab (something I am not proud of today, but it was the only option at the time), and at the Mayo Clinic in Minnesota. By 1977, we had all the pieces in place. Our goal was to perform our first open-heart procedure in a controlled environment.

We did not want to do an emergency operation as our first one. I knew that if we were to do an open-heart procedure, and the patient did not survive, it would jeopardize our program. At the time, the mortality rate from bypass surgery was around 10 to 15 percent, not the current 1 to 2 percent.

In 1977, fate intervened. I received a call at around 9 PM from Lloyd, our Mayo Clinic-trained cardiologist. He had a patient in the catheterization lab, who was in his forties and had suffered an acute heart attack at a basketball game. South Dakota was a small state, and this patient was well-known and respected there.

Lloyd informed me that the patient had a blockage of the left anterior descending coronary artery (the vessel referred to as the "widow maker"). Lloyd did not think that he would survive without an emergency operation, and it was too risky to try to transport him to the Mayo Clinic or the University of Minnesota Medical Center, which were the closest hospitals doing open-heart surgery.

"Bob, I know that we said we were not going to do an emergency operation, but if we don't operate, I believe he will die," Lloyd explained. "A large part of his heart muscle is involved. I know it's a lot to ask, but do you think we're ready to operate?"

I knew my team was prepared, but was the risk worth the reward? I was not sure; however, I was trained to save lives, and this man needed an operation even if it meant my career would be placed in harm's way. You see, if I lost the patient, all the naysayers who did not want heart surgery in South Dakota would win their argument, and cardiac care would be set back quite a while, perhaps years.

I raced to the hospital from my farm in Crooks, South Dakota, about twelve miles away. Upon arriving, I met Lloyd in the radiology reading room. He showed me the heart angiogram, films we use for predicting the need for a surgical procedure. After looking at the film, I agreed with Lloyd: we had to operate quickly or the patient would most likely die in transit to Minnesota.

My team was on ready alert 24/7 to answer their beepers for a 911 call. I called the hospital operator and told her to place that call to the surgical team. Everyone arrived within thirty minutes, from the operating room nurses to the heart-bypass technicians. Juanita, the surgical assistant whom I had brought from Michigan, had done thousands of procedures and was a great asset to have this particular day. Besides me, she was the only one with any experience doing a heart operation.

The surgery lasted six hours. By 5 AM, we had performed the first coronary bypass surgical procedure in the state of South Dakota. It was a success. I will never forget that operation. It was an exhilarating experience that the entire team would be proud of for a lifetime because they were a part of history. The patient did remarkably well and was home in seven days. He became a very dear friend of mine and a strong supporter of our program. Long after I left, that program saved countless thousands of lives and is still very prominent and active today.

Around sunrise, I walked my nurse assistant, Gail, to the parking lot. I was staying at the hospital all night to ensure that our patient's every need was met, in case something was to happen. I turned to Gail and said, "It's time for me to quit surgery."

She looked at me quizzically. "What are you talking about? You just performed the first open-heart procedure in South Dakota. Your career has just begun, and you're on top of your game. What do you mean, you have to quit?"

"I don't know how to explain it, but I just have a sense that my work here is completed. I must find out what I'm really supposed to do."

Surgery was no longer the specialty for me. I knew I had to do something different. I had to find a better way to help people.

It wouldn't be until February 1981, however, that I got serious about quitting heart surgery. Up until then, I continued to perform many more bypass operations. But sadly, many of my patients wound up back in the operating room two and three times—to undergo the same harrowing open-heart surgeries. And each time the risks were higher.

Why? Because they hadn't changed the very habits that put them there in the first place—being overweight, overworked, sedentary, smoking, and more.

I began to realize that I was doing little or nothing to make my patients healthy or younger. I was simply prolonging their deaths. I then began to see, with profound clarity, the potential of an exciting new approach to medicine that would make it possible not only to reverse coronary heart disease and other life-stealing diseases—but to prevent them from ever occurring.

In 1981, another inspiring experience happened. I became friends with George Sheehan, MD. In his book, *The Running Life,* he wrote in the front cover: "To Bob Willix, the surgeon who will eventually prove that the knife is the lesser weapon. Exercise is the new medicine."

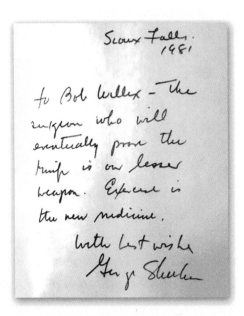

He was so right. I knew through my own workouts that exercise was the best anti-aging pill you can take. My basic mantra for anyone who wanted to prevent disease and age well became: move, move, and move.

Then came the day when I told my new surgical partner, Louis, that I was going to take a leave of absence to explore the field of medicine called preventive medicine. "I don't think I'll ever come back to the operating room."

"You love the excitement too much. You'll be back," he said. "You just need some time off."

I remember what happened next as clearly as if it were yesterday. I bundled up in warm clothing to get on my Honda Gold Wing Motorcycle. It was a beautiful, bright sunny day, about 40 degrees and not a cloud in the sky. I mounted the motorcycle like an old cowboy would mount his horse. I rode all the way to Nebraska, about sixty to eighty miles away. The ride was meditative. I pondered my future and searched my soul for answers.

On the way back to South Dakota, I stopped to visit one of the young physicians whom I had trained. She was in practice in a small town outside Sioux Falls. I asked her if I could use her telephone. I called my then-wife to inform her that I was quitting heart surgery, and we would discuss this when I came home.

As I rode that day, I knew I would never look back after that decision, and I began my pursuit of natural means to slow the aging process. I was just shy of my fortieth birthday; today, I am seventy-eight.

Everything that happened to me—from being inspired by my dad's athleticism and vibrancy to becoming a vegetarian (vegan) runner— ignited a passion in me for anything other than sawing patients open and operating on their hearts. It took about a decade, but I made the transition from a thriving surgical practice to anti-aging medicine.

I promoted lifestyle changes as aggressive and therapeutic approaches to reversing and preventing degenerative disease. Nutrition, exercise, stress reduction, and supplements became key. As I studied new developments in anti-aging medicine, I began to emphasize hormone assessment and replacement, and later telomere protection and the incorporation of natural peptides to signal the cells to revert to normal function. In my patients, the results of applying these largely natural therapies were dramatic. They were healthier. They did not require invasive interventions like surgery. They were more energetic. And, they were getting younger before my very eyes.

Because of my work with tens of thousands of patients, it became abundantly clear to me that there are distinct but interrelated causes of aging—and that if you can prevent them, then the aging process will slow down considerably, debilitating illnesses will become nonexistent, and that anyone can find a life of health, vitality, and happiness—and a long-lived one at that.

This book is about how to age slowly and successfully without life-shortening illnesses. You do it by *picking up* your nutrition, your physical activity and well-being, your body's natural healing ability, your hormones, and your internal aging regulators. When you begin living my dad's philosophy: *Let's pick it up*, you will rejuvenate your body, stay youthful, and live with abundant and vibrant health.

Aging Is Optional

I say this because there are seven causes of aging—and, more importantly, they are all under your control. Those causes are:

1. **OXIDATION AND FREE RADICAL DAMAGE**

2. **INFLAMMATION**

3. **HORMONES AND PEPTIDES**

4. **SHORTENED TELOMERES**

5. **INACTIVITY**

6. **NUTRITIONAL DEFICIENCIES**

7. **STRESS**

The Rejuvenation Solution will teach you what they are and how these *seven causes of aging* can be controlled and modified by integrating *the seven solutions for aging* in your lifestyle:

 ❶ GEROPROTECTORS:
THE NEXT GENERATION OF ANTIOXIDANTS

 ❷ INFLAMMABOTS

 ❸ THE HORMONE-PEPTIDE CONNECTION

 ❹ TELOMERASE ACTIVATORS

 ❺ MUSCLES AND THEIR ANTI-AGING GENES

 ❻ REJUVENATION NUTRITION

 ❼ AGE-DEFYING STRESS MANAGEMENT

My 7-Day Rejuvenation Plan

To put each of these synergistic solutions together, I'll give you a 7-day plan as a jump-start to get your anti-aging lifestyle going. We physicians have long known that it takes just seven days to see true physiological change in the body. Infections and acute inflammation, for example, generally clear up in a week, given the right resources.

Over a seven-day stretch, you'll take specific actions to add years to your life and slow the aging process. During this week, you'll alter your nutrition by following a seven-day meal plan, work out using an anti-aging workout, and practice meditation. I'll provide an anti-aging supplement protocol and show you how to get started on hormone replacement and peptide rejuvenation. The more of these guidelines you follow, the less you will age and the better you'll feel and look. Then simply replicate the seven-day plan, week after week, and you'll successfully fight the ravages of age—and reverse the aging process.

The Rejuvenation Solution gives you a clear understanding of how decline begins—and exactly what to do about it. You can take control over your age and look and feel younger. Using the latest in anti-aging research, my real-life experiences, and natural remedies, you'll revitalize your body in as little as seven days with these complementary, synergistic actions:

- Supplement with special geroprotectors to reverse aging—some of which have just been discovered.
- Create a body free from chronic inflammation and strengthen your immune system in the process to prevent the common diseases of aging.
- Release more anti-aging hormones and peptides into your body through natural hormone therapy, everyday foods, and other positive lifestyle actions.
- Add life and length to your telomeres with simple lifestyle changes and a few well-chosen supplements.

- Identify anti-aging, muscle-enhancing exercises that suit you best.
- Replenish your nutrient stores with key anti-aging foods that can pay huge dividends and reduce the likelihood of age-related conditions. You can actually eat yourself into a healthier, more youthful body.
- Apply ancient and modern practices to quiet your mind, heart, spirit, body, and environment—in order to activate healing and create a body, mind, and spirit that is eternally optimistic and youthful.

If you're ready, the journey back in time begins now—so let's pick it up.

OXIDATION AND FREE RADICAL DAMAGE

At this very moment, some nasty and damaging molecules are rampaging through your body, looking to puncture your cell membranes, while other protection-obsessed molecules are on their trail—like police officers hunting criminals, neutralizing and deactivating them. These processes are oxidation and anti-oxidation, respectively, a part of being alive that has to be regulated so that you don't succumb to chronic diseases and faster aging.

As for oxidation, oxygen is to blame. Yes, we need oxygen to live, but it turns out that oxygen has a dark side. Oxygen molecules can split into single atoms with unpaired electrons. These are called "free radicals" (more on this issue to follow). These can damage your cell walls and DNA and RNA inside cells—the basic building blocks of genetics. Too many free radicals cause oxidation.

Oxidation is a bit like the rusting of the chrome on my Harley. When chrome is exposed to oxygen, iron oxide, or rust, is formed. Oxidation of the human body results in similar deterioration.

So basically, oxidation occurs in our body all the time, as we process the oxygen we breathe and our cells produce energy from it.

What Are Free Radicals?

You've probably heard of free radicals before. Maybe they are a little difficult to understand. When I explain free radicals to my patients, I ask them to visualize a horde of Vikings roaming around inside your body. Imagine this army attacking and damaging healthy cells, breaking down collagen that keeps your skin firm and youthful, attacking your eyes so that you develop cataracts, wreaking havoc inside your circulatory system to cause heart disease and stroke, joining forces with air pollution and cigarette smoke (if you smoke), and so on.

Technically, unlike stable molecules, which have electrons paired so that their positive and negative electric charges cancel each other out, a free radical has an unpaired, electrically charged electron that is hungry for a mate. Free radicals do their damage by stealing electrons from stable molecules.

As a result, normal body structures break down and don't repair themselves. This free-radical chain reaction can pierce cell membranes, allowing fluids to leak out and disrupting the ability of the cells to take in nutrients. And in breaking up DNA and RNA, mutations are created that reproduce uncontrollably.

Free radicals include reactive oxygen species (ROS) and other molecules with unpaired electrons. ROS is largely responsible for slowing down cellular function, eventually leading to tissue and organ injury. Most free radical damage is caused by the reactive oxygen species.

Some free radicals serve useful purposes. For instance, your immune system relies on them to help destroy bacteria. When free radicals are generated in excess, however, they are toxic. The net result is termed "oxidative stress," or "oxidative damage." It means that the pace of free radical production is happening faster than the rate the body can create antioxidants in order to fight them. The body's antioxidant defenses are thus overwhelmed, and tissue damage occurs.

Antioxidants are substances from food, supplements, or molecules produced by the body that diffuse the damage done by oxidation and free radicals and prevent them from causing further damage. To offset and prevent aging, we must fortify our antioxidant defenses.

Anti-Aging Pioneer:
Denham Harman, MD, PhD

The "free radical theory of aging" was first proposed in the fifties by Denham Harman, professor emeritus at the University of Nebraska Medical School and founder of the American Aging Association and the International Association of Biomedical Gerontology. Harman was deeply curious about life and the aging process. "Everything dies. Why?" he once asked himself.

In 1949, he enrolled in the Stanford School of Medicine to study biology and medicine, all the while wracking his brain over why humans and animals get old. The term *free radicals* popped into his head one day, and he knew he was on to something. However, there was nothing in the scientific literature linking free radicals to aging, so Harman decided to investigate further. He first detailed his investigations in a 1954 paper titled "Free Radical Theory of Aging." In 1957, Harman tested his theory in the lab. He administered dietary antioxidants to mice and found that they prolonged the animals' life spans. Harmon suspected that taking antioxidant supplements such as beta-carotene, zinc, vitamins E and C, and a handful of other nutrients could improve both length of life as well as quality of a person's life. Thus, he proposed that we can treat aging by taking antioxidant supplements.

At the time, though, his colleagues scoffed at the theory that free radicals triggered aging and that antioxidants could prevent it. Then came the sixties, when researchers began to pay more attention to Harman's work and take seriously the notion that free radicals are involved in not only aging, but also in many diseases. Since then, many dietary antioxidant studies have been conducted over the years, confirming that free radicals do play a key role in the aging process—especially in the early stages of atherosclerosis, Alzheimer's disease, and age-related conditions like sagging skin and bone breakage. Scientists have now found that those at the highest risk of cell damage and the aging it produces are people whose diets are low in fruits, vegetables, and other high-antioxidant foods.

Today, Harman's "theory" is hardly a theory at all, but a fact of aging. It is now deemed by most scientists to be one of the most valid explanations of why we get old and sick. As for Harman, who in his eighties ran two miles a day, he lived to the amazing age of ninety-eight.

Understanding the Consequences of Oxidative Stress

As we age, our bodies cannot generate enough antioxidants to neutralize the number of free radicals that are bombarding the system each day. Over many years, accumulated oxidative damage to our tissues contributes to the aging of our body and diseases, such as cancer, diabetes, and heart disease. The ensuing result is that we produce too many ROS molecules, and the aging of cells and tissues begins to slow the organs' function. Additionally, cell repair cannot be met as fast as the cell death is occurring.

Oxidative stress also is responsible for many of the visual changes in our appearance as we age, such as wrinkles and loose, sagging skin.

One of the major aging issues with oxidation is that it creates more inflammation in the intestines. This interferes with the absorption of nutrients found in antioxidant-rich fruits and vegetables.

This oxidative stress may be either mild or severe. As more and more reports are pouring in, a lot of information is unfolding about oxidative stress in relation to several other diseases.

The table below lists the diseases caused by oxidative stress.

Diseases and Conditions Caused by Oxidative Stress

Aging Diseases

Arthritis, diabetes, osteoarthritis, cataracts, macular degeneration, prostate problems

Cancer

Cancers of the prostate, breast, lung, colon, bladder, uterus, ovaries, skin, stomach, liver, and lymphoma

Cardiovascular Diseases

Arteriosclerosis, heart failure, heart attack, kidney failure, high blood pressure, stroke, impaired circulation, bad cholesterol and plaque formation

Digestive Diseases

Inflammatory bowel disease, ulcerative colitis, Crohn's disease, gastritis, pancreatitis, and peptic ulcer

Eye, Ear, Nose, Throat, and Teeth

Cataracts, glaucoma, macular degeneration, hearing loss, ear infections, sinusitis, periodontal (gum) disease, nose, mouth and throat (upper respiratory tract) disease

Exercise and Athletic Performance

Overtraining syndrome and compromised immunity

Infectious Diseases and Immunology

Viral infections, common cold, bacterial infection, chronic fatigue syndrome

Kidney Failure and Dialysis
Kidney failure, renal toxicity, oxidative stress from dialysis

Liver Diseases
Hepatitis, cirrhosis

Lung Diseases
Asthma, pneumonia, bronchitis (chronic and acute), adult respiratory distress syndrome (ARDS)

Male Problems
Prostate enlargement, prostate cancer, balding and hair loss, male infertility

Neurodegenerative Diseases
Parkinson's disease, Alzheimer's disease, multiple sclerosis, dementia, Huntington's disease

Pregnancy, Lactation, and Childbirth Issues
Pre-eclampsia, eclampsia, hypertension, gestational diabetes, immune problems in newborns

Skin Disorders
Psoriasis, eczema, SLE (lupus), vasculitis, atopic dermatitis, contact dermatitis, seborrheic dermatitis, acne, UV radiation skin damage

What Triggers Oxidative Stress?

When you're familiar with what triggers oxidative stress and its resulting diseases, you can better avoid and prevent it. In addition to natural processes, such as aging, oxidative stress comes from UV rays due to sun exposure, tobacco and smoking, excess alcohol consumption, certain foods, and toxins in our environment or even in your skin-care products. Let me elaborate.

If you stay out in the sun too long unprotected, the exposure creates free radicals and damages DNA. Damaged DNA causes mutations that result in skin cancer.

Free radicals from sun exposure also weaken elastin fibers—your skin's "rubber bands"—and damaged elastin makes your skin sag. Free radicals generated from prolonged sun exposure also destroy collagen, weakening the skin's structural support. Your skin gets thin and crepey. Wrinkles then appear and refuse to disappear. Protecting yourself against excessive sun exposure keeps oxidative skin damage to a minimum and preserves your skin's health and beauty.

Smoking has been shown to increase free radicals and oxidative stress. A Surgeon General report notes that "massive amounts of free radicals in cigarette smoke cause inflammation and oxidative stress, which damages cells, tissues, and organs." The report concluded that "there is no safe level of exposure to cigarette smoke."

Germs, including bacteria, viruses, and fungi, also inflict oxidative injury and disease.

Certain foods contribute to high levels of free radicals in the body. Many of these are processed foods that have been changed from their original form before they reach your table. These "processes" typically include adding some nutrients while removing others and adding questionable preservatives to sustain freshness.

Sugary foods also generate free radicals and trigger oxidative stress. The result of this process is glycation, a reaction in which sugar binds with proteins and damages cells throughout the human body. Glycation produces accelerated glycation end products (AGEs), which are sticky, gooey proteins that coat cells in such a way that each cell looks like a candy-coated apple. Cells become rigid and unable to function normally. The process promotes skin wrinkles, fatigue, mental decline, heart problems, and other age-related illnesses.

There is also a reduction in the number of immune system cells with glycation. As a result, the immune system itself cannot protect the body from even simple invasions from viruses or bacteria. Certain cells can mutate into cancer cells and grow without restraint.

Besides sugar, other big dietary offenders are white rice, potatoes, pasta, and bread, which all cause oxidation because of their *glycemic* content—meaning that they dangerously elevate sugar in the body.

Like some foods, alcoholic beverages trigger oxidative stress by increasing free radicals in the body. They also inflict indirect oxidative stress by damaging your liver. This means your liver function is impaired; it has a hard time filtering free radicals and other toxins from the body. Alcohol also reduces the levels of antioxidants in your body.

Many people use skin creams to fight or mask the visible signs of aging. Yet what they don't know is that many of these products contain high levels of additives, which are basically allergens that can increase free radicals. These allergens incite your immune system to recruit inflammatory cells to your skin that act to fight off the offending additive. The immune cells release toxic chemicals in the process—and these toxic chemicals increase oxidative stress. The additives themselves are directly toxic to skin cells. You have to be very careful about what you apply to your skin.

Mitochondrial Oxidation Is Linked to Aging

If you're looking for ways to not only stay healthy but also to lengthen your life, look no further than your mitochondria. Found in every cell of the human body except red blood cells, the mitochondria are little energy factories that keep everything powered and functioning. If these factories are not operating well, then the parts of your body that require the most power begin to falter. I'm talking mainly about your brain, heart, muscles, liver, and kidneys.

Under healthy conditions, the mitochondria take in nutrients, break them down, and create energy-rich molecules for the cell. There is growing evidence that by taking care of them and keeping them healthy, you might live longer.

Mitochondria

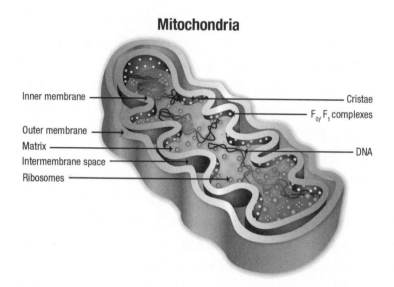

Inner membrane
Outer membrane
Matrix
Intermembrane space
Ribosomes

Cristae
F_{0}, F_{1} complexes

DNA

A review article published in 2016 in *Molecular Cell* pointed out that mitochondria contribute to specific aspects of the aging process. These include:

Cellular senescence. This is a state in which cells can no longer divide. Many studies show that ROS can induce cellular senescence, which leads to mitochondrial oxidative stress and ultimately aging.

Chronic inflammation. One of the hallmarks of aging is the development of a chronic, inflammatory state often called "inflammaging" (see chapter 3). It harms immunity and is a known risk factor for premature death in the elderly. Scientists have discovered that when mitochondrial function is compromised, inflammation is likely to be triggered and the immune system is weakened.

Age-dependent decline in stem cell activity. Adult stem cells are those that maintain our tissues and differentiate into the cell types that make up the tissue in which they reside. Stem cells also have the ability to self-renew. However, these processes become less efficient over time, as mitochondrial DNA can be damaged (see text to follow). This impairs the function of the mitochondria, and consequently, adult stem cell function. The self-renewal ability of stem cells declines, too.

One of the main issues here is the fact that the mitochondria also happen to be the main generating source of free radicals. This is because 85 to 90 percent of cellular oxygen consumption occurs in these structures. That is quite a bit of oxygen use, and it does generate oxidation. When oxidation damages the mitochondrial membranes (walls) directly, the mitochondria might produce even more free radicals. It's quite a vicious cycle. There is obviously quite a cumulative impact of oxidative stress on mitochondrial DNA, in particular. This may be responsible for many age-associated diseases and disorders, such as heart disease and neurodegenerative disorders like Alzheimer's.

So it seems that mitochondria play an important part in aging. By rejuvenating mitochondrial function or improving mitochondrial quality and decreasing oxidative stress, you can help support mitochondrial health and slow down, or even reverse, the rate at which you age.

Fortunately, the body can produce natural antioxidants to combat the negative effects of oxidation in the mitochondria and in the body as a whole. We can also eat more foods rich in antioxidants, supplement with antioxidants, and get adequate exercise. These strategies are important because as we age, the number of antioxidants produced by the body decreases.

ASK DR. BOB: Does calorie restriction really fight aging?

Caloric restriction is a great way to improve mitochondrial function and increase longevity. The easiest way to do this is through a strategy called "intermittent fasting." Generally, you fast overnight (while sleeping) and do not eat again for fourteen to sixteen hours. Thus, if your last meal in the evening ends at 7 PM, you would not eat again until 9 AM or 11 AM the next day—and confine your meals to an eight-hour eating window. When you do this, you reduce mitochondrial free radical production.

Antioxidants to the Rescue

To counter oxidative stress and the impact of free radicals, the body is endowed with compounds called antioxidants. These antioxidants are produced either endogenously (within the body) or received from exogenous sources (outside the body).

Important endogenous antioxidants include enzymes. They take free radicals apart and render them helpless. There are three major enzymes involved. Superoxide dismutase (SOD) focuses on defusing the master free radical, superoxide. Catalase specializes in disarming hydrogen peroxide and the lipid (fatty) peroxides that are generated by cell membranes. Glutathione peroxidase also stops the hydrogen peroxide radical by converting it into oxygen and water.

To function properly, these enzymes require certain antioxidant minerals like selenium, manganese, copper, and zinc, and exogenous sources of antioxidant vitamins like vitamin A, C, E, and beta carotene. Other compounds with antioxidant activity include glutathione and flavonoids, among others.

Vitamin C is a well-known and potent antioxidant. Although many animals can manufacture vitamin C, humans cannot make this vitamin; we must obtain it from food.

As we age, the number of antioxidants produced by the body decreases, which is why many medical experts recommend adding foods rich in antioxidants, along with supplements, to the diet.

Nutrient antioxidants work by a sacrificial mode. For example, vitamin E can attach itself to a free radical and neutralize it so that it can't do any damage. However, sometimes in this process, vitamin E becomes a free radical. When this happens, the molecule that results is a reactive oxygen species (ROS).

Even spices exert antioxidant activity. One is turmeric, which contains curcumin, a powerful antioxidant. It can deliver a one-two punch against free radicals: neutralizing them and stimulating the body's own antioxidant enzymes.

Then there is sulforaphane, a chemical in broccoli. It boosts antioxidant enzymes in the lungs that offer protection against the onslaught of free radicals from polluted air, pollen, diesel exhaust, tobacco smoke, and other toxins we breathe in.

Antioxidants at Work in Your Cells

The diagram to follow shows a typical cell with its various organelles and other structures, and the specific antioxidants that protect them:

- *Nucleus:* Working as the cell's control center, the nucleus contains genes. It regulates the cell's growth and reproduction.
- *Protective antioxidant:* Vitamin E.
- *Mitochondria:* This is the energy factory of the cell.
- *Protective antioxidants:* Vitamin E, glutathione, glutathione peroxidase (an important antioxidant enzyme), SOD, and manganese.
- *Endoplasmic reticulum:* Connected to the nucleus, this organelle functions as a manufacturing and packaging system, transporting proteins through the cell.
- *Protective antioxidant:* Beta-carotene.
- *Cytoplasm:* This is a gel-like substance that fills the cell, supporting the cell's organelles, transporting genetic material within the cell, and protecting the cell's organelles and genetic material from damage.
- *Protective antioxidants:* Copper, zinc, vitamin C, glutathione, glutathione peroxidase, and SOD.

- **Lysosome:** This structure holds enzymes that were created by the cell. Its job is to digest food or break down the cell when it dies off.
- **Protective antioxidants:** Vitamin E, vitamin C, and beta-carotene.
- **Peroxisomes:** Most abundant in the liver and kidney, peroxisomes absorb nutrients that the cell has acquired to digest fatty acids. The enzyme in peroxisomes is called peroxidase.
- **Protective antioxidant:** Catalase (a very important enzyme for protecting the cell from oxidative stress).
- **Lipid bilayer:** This is a dual layer of lipids that form the cell's membrane, or wall. It maintains the shape of a cell and helps decide what can enter the cell. Therefore, it is vital for the survival and function of the cell.
- **Protective antioxidants:** Vitamin E and beta-carotene.

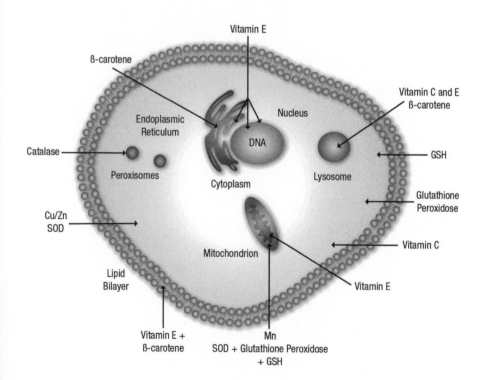

To sum up: All antioxidants and antioxidant enzymes prevent cell damage linked to the development of degenerative, aging conditions, such as heart disease; cataracts; Alzheimer's, Lou Gehrig's, and Parkinson's diseases; and cancers. Antioxidants bolster your immune system and slow down the aging process.

So, yes, many people are growing older and weaker, slowly rusting away like a scrapyard of abandoned Harleys. But you don't have to be one of them. The good news is that *geroprotectors*, the exogenous (outside the body) antioxidants are available to boost the body's internal system as you get older. Keep turning the page to find out about how this next generation of antioxidants can *turn back the clock*.

Solution:

GEROPROTECTORS— THE NEXT GENERATION OF ANTIOXIDANTS

H. L. was fifty-three years old when he first came to my office. A former athlete, he was referred by a friend because I was an athlete, too, and he did not want to stop exercising. Several other doctors had told him, "Just stop exercising."

His chief complaints were insomnia and low attention span, for which he had been taking the prescription drug Adderall for quite a long time. He also suffered from chronic constipation and irritable colon, frequent night-time urination, difficulty breathing, and high triglycerides in his blood. He was seeing a cardiologist, a pulmonary specialist, a gastroenterologist, and a family doctor. H. L. told me he thought he was healthy.

Does he sound healthy to you? It amazes me how we view health as the lack of a clear disease. The cardiologist alerted him about his family history of heart disease. The pulmonologist told him he had low lung capacity. The gastroenterologist had scheduled him for a CT scan of his intestines to see what was wrong.

On his initial visit with me, he weighed 235 pounds on a six-foot, four-inch frame and had a body fat percentage of 29. After my exam, I determined that he had a lot of oxidative stress from his high-pressure job and from his poor nutrition alone. I asked him to let me test to see if he truly was at risk of heart disease. I used a VO2 test—an evaluation I've done for the past thirty-six years on most of my patients. It determines levels of health of their cardiovascular system, as well as their lung capacity and their leg strength.

Clinically, this test is very helpful in determining risk of heart disease, along with fitness status and cardiac output. I call this test "the best kept secret in medicine" because most physicians cannot even interpret the test, let alone know how valuable it is.

H. L.'s VO2 results immediately told me he was at a very low risk for heart disease, despite his high triglycerides and cholesterol. His lung capacity revealed that he did have lung problems, however. His CT scan reported diverticulosis (pouches in the large intestine) but was otherwise normal.

Another major finding was that a crucial enzyme in his body, MAOB (monomine oxidase B) was not working to its fullest capacity. The normal function of this enzyme is to assist in the breakdown of the neurotransmitters dopamine, epinephrine, norepinephrine, and serotonin. Faulty MAOB can result in diseases of aging, including Parkinson's disease, Alzheimer's disease, and changes in mental capacity.

All of his tests pointed to oxidation being a factor in his health. Because oxidation has such a strong nutritional component, I altered his nutrition significantly to a plant-based plan, supported by supplementation.

I removed all oxidizing foods from his diet: rice, potatoes, pasta, bread, alcohol, and high-amine foods such as aged, pickled, or marinated meat and beef; most kinds of pork; most cheeses (except cottage or ricotta); yogurt;

and chocolate. Foods contain one or more compounds called amines, which are formed by the breakdown of proteins in foods high in certain amino acids. Reducing high-amine foods in the diet may help people with an MAOB enzyme deficiency by preventing a neurotransmitter buildup.

I supplemented his nutrition with three main products: clary sage oil, a supplement high in antioxidants; omega-3 fatty acids from a plant source; and an Ayurvedic herbal formulation containing thirty-four different herbs, all of which have antioxidant and adaptogenic (stress-resisting) properties.

As a result of this approach, his insomnia was relieved, he lost seventeen pounds in six weeks, and his chronic digestive problems disappeared. Further, he became more mentally alert and stopped taking the Adderall for his ADD symptoms. His energy soared so much that he increased his cardiovascular training, and he now works out very intensely five to six times a week.

As a footnote, H. L. related to me last month that he had a glass of wine one evening. When he went to exercise the next day, he could not get through his workout because he was too fatigued. I told him that alcohol was toxic to his system in part because the MAOB enzyme is impaired by alcohol. This is a common problem among people who have a defective MAOB SNP (single nucleotide peptide).

As I told H. L., despite what many medical experts say, alcohol is not good for you. Short term, it will slow you down and make you feel sluggish. With long-term use, it will age you because it accelerates the aging processes in the body, including oxidation, glycation, and inflammation, especially the latter.

The body can handle a great deal of the oxidative threats until we reach our twenties. Then, the free radicals increase, coupled with lifestyle choices, stress, and slowing of our internal production of antioxidants, and the result is aging. We can, however, strengthen our defenses through lifestyle and consume supplements to add protection.

Here are my geroprotector solutions for reversing oxidation and aging.

Make High-Antioxidant Food Choices

Most antioxidants are found in fruits and vegetables, as well as in spices and herbal sources such as garlic, black pepper, certain mushrooms like shiitake, curcumin, licorice, ginger, as well as many others. A plant-rich diet is one of the most powerful antioxidant defenses you can pursue. The more vegetables you eat on a daily basis, the more protection against aging you'll receive.

Let me add that some foods are higher in antioxidants than others, according to an analysis called ORAC (oxygen radical absorbance capacity). According to ORAC, the top five fruits are prunes (dried plums), cranberries, blackberries, raspberries, and strawberries. Kale, spinach, Brussels sprouts, alfalfa sprouts, and broccoli scored highest among vegetables. Eat as many of these foods as you can each week.

Take Geroprotector Supplements

There are many good antioxidants, but you cannot possibly take them all. I've carefully compiled a list of the best newly researched antioxidants and anti-aging molecules out there—which I call geroprotectors. They work best when you follow a high-antioxidant nutrition plan. Several of these supplements come from the practice of Ayurveda that prescribes plants or their components and extracts to fight against aging and illness.

Alpha-Lipoic Acid (ALA)

What is it? The most unique of all antioxidants, ALA does things other antioxidants can't do, such as working in both watery and fatty parts of the body. It can thus get to all parts of your cells to zap free radicals. Further, alpha-lipoic acid can cross the blood-brain barrier to protect against brain diseases like Alzheimer's and other forms of dementia.

Unique properties: ALA lengthens your telomeres (shorter telomeres mean shorter life). Telomeres are found on the tips of chromosomes and are critical in controlling the aging process. (See chapter 8 for more information.)

ALA also regenerates glutathione, your body's "master" antioxidant. It keeps all other antioxidants performing at peak levels and is the body's most potent antioxidant.

ALA has many other benefits. It:

- Helps treat type 2 diabetes, especially diabetic nerve damage (peripheral neuropathy).
- Can repair a damaged and scarred liver.
- May help prevent cancer by triggering mitochondrial respiration that induces the death of cancer cells. Oncologists do not use ALA, however, because they want the damaging effect of chemotherapy, namely oxidative stress, and ALA prevents this effect. This has always baffled me!
- Can help eliminate some side effects of chemotherapy, including the restoration and conduction of nerve cells.

Recommended dosage: 600 to 1,200 milligrams daily. Therapeutically, ALA is most effective when given intravenously at 1,500 to 2,000 milligrams daily.

Astaxanthin

What is it? Derived from algae, this potent antioxidant is also a collagen *hydrolysate*, a type of protein high in the amino acids glycine and proline. After you reach the age of twenty-five, the body's natural ability to produce these amino acids diminishes, but they can be easily replenished through supplementation. As a plant-based geroprotector, astaxanthin is fat soluble. This means that it can enter the fatty membranes of cells very easily.

Unique properties: Astaxanthin doubles the action of a rejuvenation gene called FOXO3. What's more, it revs up a cell's ability to cope with damaged proteins, a marker of aging in many tissues.

Astaxanthin also:

- Helps prevent and treat oxidative stress and inflammation without triggering the potential gastrointestinal bleeding seen with NSAIDs or steroids, such as prednisone.
- Protects DNA.
- Guards the body against damage from UV radiation light.
- Is one of the most powerful free-radical attackers among antioxidants.

Dosage: 4 to 12 milligrams daily.

Glutathione (GSH)

What is it? Glutathione is one of the most important antioxidants in the human body. It is also a *tripeptide*, comprised largely of three amino acids: glutamine, glycine, and cysteine—a chain that regulates enzyme systems in the body. (I talk about peptides in detail in chapter 3.)

Glutathione levels in the body may be compromised by a number of factors, including poor nutrition, environmental toxins, advancing age and stress.

Unique properties: Boosting glutathione levels in your body may provide many health benefits.

Glutathione:

- Reduces cell damage in alcoholic and nonalcoholic fatty liver disease.
- Improves the body's use of insulin.
- Increases mobility for people with peripheral artery disease (clogged arteries in the limbs).

- Eases symptoms of Parkinson's disease.
- May alleviate respiratory disease symptoms.

Dosage: Taking glutathione by mouth has not been shown in research to have much of a benefit. It is better to supplement with glutathione intravenously. In my clinic, we give glutathione drips of 2000 to 4000 milligrams. For anti-aging, we follow that with hyperbaric oxygen and have seen excellent results.

The Power of Intravenous (IV) Nutrient Therapy

An effective way to receive antioxidant therapy is through IV nutrient therapy. Administered through an IV drip, vitamins, minerals, amino acids, antioxidants, anti-aging compounds, and other nutrients are delivered to the body directly through the bloodstream slowly over a period of time, usually thirty to forty-five minutes, depending on the nutrients used.

Traditionally offered in hospital settings, IV drips are now available in spas, doctors' offices, and special stand-alone clinics. They are used to treat an array of health conditions, including aging, lowered immunity, migraines, toxicities, fatigue, skin conditions, weight problems, and more.

IV nutrient therapy is not a fad but real medicine, firmly based on medical evidence. Research shows that this targeted nutrition boost can help in the prevention and treatment of a variety of diseases and conditions and improve your general health.

At my clinic, for example, we administer glutathione drips, high-dose vitamin C IVs, alpha lipoic acid drips, and "cocktails" that combine these nutrients. We also offer chelation therapy using EDTA, a man-made amino acid that binds to heavy metals to remove them from the body. It also functions as an antioxidant, helps prevent heart disease, and increases blood flow to organs. EDTA chelation involves a series of IV drips (thirty or more), lasting three to four hours each. It is very effective in treating and preventing heart disease and resolving heavy metals toxicity, though not widely accepted by conventional medicine.

Beyond the restoration of nutrients and overall rejuvenation, I feel that IV nutrient therapy may one day be used more widely as adjunctive therapy for cancer patients rather than destroying the immune system with chemotherapy.

L-Citrulline

What is it? L-citrulline is a nonessential amino acid, rarely found in food, but highly concentrated in beetroot, garlic, pomegranate, and dark chocolate. It is very commonly used among weight lifters to build muscle mass when combined with arginine.

Unique properties: As an anti-aging compound, citrulline stimulates muscle protein synthesis (MPS), or muscle growth in the elderly, who typically experience muscle loss (sarcopenia) and have a difficult time gaining muscle.

L-citrulline is a unique amino acid in that it exerts its effects on heart health as an antioxidant to prevent free radical formation in the smooth muscles of the heart. Further, it boosts nitric oxide (NO) production in the body. NO helps your arteries relax and work better, improving blood flow throughout your body and protecting the walls of your blood vessels. This helps treat or prevent many diseases.

Dosage: 3 to 6 grams taken with 1500 milligrams to 3 grams of arginine.

Coenzyme Q10 (CoQ10)

What is it? This antioxidant occurs naturally in the body as ubiquinone but its level declines with aging. CoQ10 is also in many foods, including fish and organ meats (which I do not recommend), but there is plenty in legumes, soybeans, strawberries, lentils, spinach, cauliflower, seaweed, and algae.

Chlorophyll (the green pigment in plants) and sunlight boosts the CoQ10 production in the body. If you combine green leafy vegetables with prudent exposure to sunlight, you can supercharge your body's own CoQ10 production.

Unique properties: CoQ10 increases levels of key anti-aging enzymes called sirtuins to promote longevity. Sirtuins, specifically SIRT1 and SIRT3, are intimately related to longevity through their ability to turn off aging genes. By activating these sirtuins, you gain control over one of your body's anti-aging "switches."

CoQ10 also:

- Confers health benefits in elderly people by preventing chronic oxidative stress associated with cardiovascular and neurode-generative diseases.
- Protects against muscle loss that occurs with aging.
- Serves as a natural defense mechanism for every cell in the body.
- Helps lower blood pressure.
- Offers neurogenic protection for anyone with heavy metal toxicity.

Dosage: 200 to 400 milligrams daily. If you're taking statins or have known heart disease, high blood pressure, or cancer, take 400 to 800 milligrams daily. Use a gel cap supplement, not a powdered one. I frequently measure CoQ10 in the blood of my patients and like to keep their levels at twice the norm because of the supplement's ability to protect the heart and rejuvenate the mitochondria.

Curcumin/Turmeric

What is it? Curcumin is the active compound in the Indian spice turmeric. It is a powerful anti-inflammatory and is a very strong antioxidant. Curcumin is also fat soluble, so it enters the fatty membrane of cells easily.

Unique properties: Curcumin switches off inflammation through its antioxidant activity. In skin cells, it physically stops inflammation so the cells don't age or rapidly degrade into cancer cells if attacked by free radicals or UV light. In clinical trials, turmeric prevents certain diseases of aging, including heart disease and liver diseases and even reverses Alzheimer's disease by preventing and removing the beta-amyloid plaque build-up in the brain.

Dosage: While there is no official consensus on effective turmeric or curcumin doses, the following have been used in research with promising results:

For osteoarthritis: 500 milligrams of turmeric extract twice daily for two or three months.

For high cholesterol: 700 milligrams of turmeric extract twice daily for three months.

For itchy skin: 500 milligrams of turmeric three times daily for two months.

ASK DR. BOB: Can I do something to prevent the flu, other than taking flu shots yearly?

I do not recommend flu shots except perhaps for the very young or elderly who are immune deficient. Rather than resort to flu shots if you are healthy, try the following regimen during flu season. I have used it for thirty-five years.

- Vitamin C in ester form: 8 to 15 grams daily.
- Goldenseal (whole herb): 250 to 500 milligrams, 4 times daily.
- Whole garlic (pressed): 3 to 4 cloves or 2,400 milligrams daily of aged garlic extract (see page 44).
- A sauté of shiitake mushrooms with onion and spinach in olive oil; add this mixture to soup or other foods at least once a day. Continue this for three to five days after the symptoms have completely been abated.

- Stay well hydrated. Drink at least eight 8-ounce glasses of distilled or filtered alkaline water (with a pH of 8.0 or higher.) Alkaline water contains many mineral antioxidants and has been shown in research to increase health and well-being.

Green Tea Extract/EGCG

What is it? Epigallocatechin-3-gallate (EGCG) is the chief antioxidant in green tea, representing 200 to 300 milligrams in a brewed cup of green tea.

Unique properties: I recommend EGCG because of its potential to lengthen telomeres. EGCG has been demonstrated in numerous studies to reduce aging, especially when you drink three cups a day on average. EGCG also:

- Protects normal cells from cancer.
- Keeps cancerous cells from multiplying and constricts blood vessels that feed tumors.
- Lowers LDL cholesterol in people with heart disease, and makes abnormal clots less likely to form.

Dosage: For optimum absorption, scientists have discovered that you should take one oral dose in the morning at least thirty minutes before breakfast, a second dose in the afternoon after not eating for at least four hours, and at least thirty minutes before dinner.

Quercetin

What is it? Abundant in many fruits and vegetables, including grapes, blueberries, cherries, onions, apples, and broccoli, quercetin is a powerful anti-aging molecule. It has more than six times the antioxidant capacity than vitamin C.

Unique properties: Quercetin is also a strong anti-inflammatory. Its antioxidant and anti-inflammatory properties may contribute to the anti-aging effect of quercetin since chronic oxidative stress and inflammation are believed to play important roles in triggering advanced aging. Quercetin also stimulates autophagy in cells—a regenerative, anti-aging process by which your body cleans out cellular debris, including toxins, and recycles damaged cell components

Dosage: 100 to 250 mg of quercetin three times a day.

Resveratrol

What is it? Resveratrol is a molecule produced in plants (such as red-wine grapes). It is part of a group of compounds called polyphenols, believed to act like antioxidants, protecting your body against damage that can put you at a greater risk for things like cancer and heart disease.

Unique properties: Resveratrol induces autophagy. It also increases levels of key anti-aging enzymes (sirtuins) that enhance longevity.

Worth noting: About twenty years ago, scientists observed a phenomenon they dubbed the French Paradox, in which the French people who eat a diet high in saturated fat and drink red wine regularly have a lower incidence of coronary heart disease and longer life span. Since the discovery that red wine contains significant amounts of resveratrol, it has led to speculation that resveratrol might confer the health benefits of drinking red wine—and explain the mystery of the French Paradox.

Dosage: 250 to 1,000 milligrams daily.

Vitamin C

What is it? Vitamin C is a powerful antioxidant, and at high doses, it prevents healthy cells from dying off. It also puts a halt to *glycation*, an aging process that involves the abnormal linking together of proteins and sugars in the body.

Unique properties: Vitamin C continues to be an anti-aging superstar.

It:

- Prevents free radicals from being cancerous or accelerating the aging process.
- Protects and strengthens the skin by boosting collagen production.
- May help prevent and treat ultraviolet (UV)-induced photo damage.
- Boosts wound healing.
- Reduces body-wide chronic inflammation.

Dosage: Although touted as an anti-aging nutrient for a long time, we now know exactly how much to take daily to halt aging (around 1,250–5,000 milligrams).

Anti-Aging Pioneer: Linus Pauling, PhD

In addition to Denham Harman, another expert in the field of antioxidants was Linus Pauling, PhD. He is best known for his research on the antioxidant vitamin C (ascorbic acid). Fascinated with its possibilities, he began analyzing the scientific and medical literature for experimental and clinical evidence as to its importance. From this research, published studies, and from his and his wife's own experiences, Pauling became convinced of the value of vitamin C in large doses to treat the common cold. In 1970, he wrote the book *Vitamin C and the Common Cold,* which became a bestseller and brought wide public attention to the vitamin, creating a huge demand for vitamin C supplements.

Later, Pauling suggested that vitamin C had value in combating the flu, cancer, cardiovascular disease, infections, and degenerative problems in the aging process. It is believed that he took around 20 grams, or 20,000 milligrams of vitamin C daily. He added other nutrients, such as vitamin E and the B vitamins, to his list of helpful supplements and published two other popular books and a number of papers, both scientific and popular, on nutritional therapy.

Pauling gave us more insight than anyone into the value of antioxidant therapy to treat disease. He was dismissed, however, by the medical community because he was a biochemist. What many people don't know is that he actually described the molecular structure of proteins and a triple fold of polypeptides before Watson and Crick identified the double-stranded DNA molecule. He really should be credited with providing the basis for their discovery.

Pauling is the only person ever to receive two unshared Nobel Prizes: for chemistry in 1954 and for peace in 1962 (for his work promoting nuclear disarmament).

Aged Garlic Extract

What is it? This supplement is created by aging garlic in diluted alcohol, without heat. The process produces unique and potent compounds—including S-allylcysteine and other S-allyl compounds. All are sulfur-based and have powerful oxidant-reducing qualities. Aged garlic extract is one of the five herbs that I would take if I were stranded on a desert island. The others include licorice root, turmeric, ginger, and golden seal.

Unique properties: Aged garlic extract has many anti-aging benefits. This supplement:

- Lowers inflammation, as seen in markers like C-reactive protein (CRP), LDL cholesterol, and high blood pressure.
- Protects against plaque formation in the heart vessels. It also reduces the size of existing plaque after only one year of daily use.
- Decreases the formation of advanced glycation end products.
- Protects the mitochondria and slows down mitochondrial DNA mutations.
- Reduces inflammation in immune cells in the brain.

- Inhibits sun damage, prevents aging at the cellular level, and prevents the formation of radical oxygen species.
- Lowers C-reactive protein by 39 percent.
- Regulates tumor necrosis factor alpha (TNF-alpha) in the liver by 35 percent. TNF ramps up the response of immune cells to a foreign object, especially to the presence of any cancerous tumors. It also promotes inflammation and can help cells heal.
- Reduces the action of thromboxane B2 (TXB2) by 33 percent, an enzyme involved in inflammation.

Garlic, in general, is an anti-bacterial, anti-fungal, and anti-parasitic agent. Aging garlic has all of these benefits, as well as some that may be unique to aging with alcohol.

Dosage: For hardening of the arteries: 250 milligrams taken daily.

For diabetes: 600 to 1,500 milligrams daily.

For high cholesterol: 1,000 to 7,200 milligrams daily in divided doses.

For high blood pressure: 960 to 7,200 milligrams, taken daily in up to three divided doses.

Geroprotective Lifestyle Strategies

In addition to eating foods rich in antioxidants and taking geroprotectors, there are important lifestyle changes you can make to reduce oxidative damage and reverse aging. For example:

- Avoid too much exposure to radiation, particularly from computers, cell phones, and sunlight.
- Balance your exercise activities. Include aerobic activity, weight training, flexibility work, and core strengthening.
- Laugh often and much. Research by Norman Cousins in the 1980s proved laughter reduces oxidative stress.
- Meditate and relax. Meditation or some form of relaxation therapy improves the production of endogenous antioxidants

like glutathione peroxidase and catalase and lowers the damage from ROS. Meditators live longer, more productive lives than non-meditators, according to new research.

- Talk to your doctor about reducing prescription drugs. The average American male over the age of sixty-five in the US is taking an average of six to eight prescription drugs. Too many prescription drugs react against each other and can depress the production of antioxidants.

ASK DR. BOB: Can my antioxidant levels be measured?

Yes, there are blood tests that measure cell levels of glutathione, CoQ10, vitamins C, A, E and total antioxidants. One such test is from SpectraCell Laboratories.

3

INFLAMMATION

What does an aching muscle, a fever, or the swelling around a cut or wound have to do with your risk of premature aging or developing diseases of aging like Alzheimer's disease or heart disease?

Plenty, as it turns out. As scientists delve deeper into aging and its causes, they have discovered that it is very much linked to *inflammation*, the same process that eases muscle soreness, resolves a fever, or heals a wound.

Under normal conditions, inflammation is a lifesaver that enables our bodies to fight off various disease-causing bacteria, viruses, and other germs. The moment any of these harmful pathogens invade the body, the process of inflammation marshals an amazing defensive attack. A type of white blood cell called mast cells give off a chemical called histamine. It makes capillaries permeable so that tiny amounts of plasma can seep out, slowing down the invaders and preparing the way for other immune defenders to enter. Another group of Pac-Man-like cells called macrophages engulf and consume the unwelcome invaders. Armies of other immune cells arrive in waves, destroying the germs and damaged tissue. Then just as quickly, inflammation subsides and healing begins. This is the positive and necessary part of the inflammatory system.

Once the invaders are compromised, the immune battalion starts to heal damaged cells, or if the attacked cells were too badly damaged, it puts them to rest. (This sort of cell death is not to be confused with apoptosis, a naturally occurring process in the body, in which cells that become damaged commit suicide in order to avoid causing harm to other cells.)

When Inflammation Becomes Chronic

But sometimes, the whole inflammation process doesn't stop on cue. The reason might be a genetic problem or issues like smoking or a poor diet. Whatever the reason, inflammation turns chronic rather than transitory. When this happens, the body can turn on itself—with results that underlie many diseases.

Diseases Caused by Chronic Inflammation

When no one was talking about it, I knew forty years ago that uncontrolled, invisible inflammation is a key villain in the development of many chronic diseases. Now scientists have just caught up to this fact, and they call the phenomenon "inflamm-aging." Chronic inflammation underlies the following diseases:

Alzheimer's disease

Asthma

Cancer

Celiac disease

Crohn's disease

Diabetes, type 2

Eczema

Fibromyalgia

Heart disease

Hepatitis (chronic and acute)

Irritable bowel syndrome

Kidney disease

Lupus

Multiple sclerosis

Osteoarthritis

Peptic ulcers

Periodontal disease

Rheumatoid arthritis

Stroke

Ulcerative colitis

Staying youthful and ageless will always be associated with less disease. But if you have inflammation-related illnesses, this is an indication that your body is aging faster than it needs to.

Chronic Inflammation and Aging

All the components of the aging process are interrelated. Excessive oxidation, for example, leads to inflammation. Inflammation, in turn, shortens telomeres at the ends of our chromosomes, and shortened telomeres lead to a shortened life span. Inflammation also imbalances many hormones involved in the aging process. If you're under persistent stress, stress hormones like cortisol and adrenaline remain too high, damaging organs. Your heart beats faster, your body temperature goes up, and blood flow to organs is impeded.

The net effect of these stress reactions is to tax the entire endocrine (hormonal) system. Both the thyroid and pituitary glands respond by reducing levels of anti-aging hormones in the body—such as estrogen, testosterone, and growth hormone. Even insulin is affected to the point that it has trouble doing its job of ushering glucose into cells for energy. If that's not enough, inflammation damages mitochondrial DNA, which then mutates and can no longer do its repair duties.

Associated with these problems is that a process called methylation. It is a simple biochemical process that occurs when one molecule hands over a methyl group, which is a carbon atom linked to three hydrogens, to another molecule. This reaction is necessary to manufacture key substances in the body such as CoQ10 and melatonin. Methylation also regulates the activity of the cardiovascular, neurological, reproductive, and detoxification systems; it is thus vital to health and anti-aging.

So you see, chronic inflammation can age you faster than you realize. If you can stop it, you can go a long way toward slowing down aging. The first step in that direction is understanding what causes chronic inflammation.

Pioneer in Anti-Aging: Rudolf Virchow

In the nineteenth century, German pathologist Rudolf Virchow was the first to observe the cellular nature of an inflammatory response. He described inflammation as a disease-causing process involving the excessive inflow and proliferation of cells caused by the release of nutrients from damaged blood vessels. It was also Virchow who suggested a link between inflammation and subsequent cancer development, after he noted the presence of white blood cells in malignant tissue. This hypothesis has recently been corroborated by numerous studies and may have therapeutic consequences.

Virchow also believed that inflammation was responsible for cardiovascular disease, diabetes, pulmonary disease, neurological disease and other chronic diseases. Extensive research within the last three decades has confirmed these observations.

What Triggers Chronic Inflammation?

Accelerated inflammation has a great deal to do with "epigenetics"—external modifications to DNA that turn genes on or off. What you eat, where you live, who you socialize with, how you think, when you sleep, whether you exercise, and how youthful you stay—all of these can eventually stimulate chemical changes to the genes that will switch them on or off over time. Additionally, in certain diseases such as cancer or Alzheimer's, various genes can be switched from operating in the normal/healthy state to one of disease.

Here's an analogy that will help you better understand epigenetics, as explained in Nessa Carey's *Epigenetics Revolution*:

Think of your entire life like a feature film. The cells in your body are the actors and actresses, essential units that make up the movie. DNA, in turn, is the script—words for the players in the film to speak. Genes would be the instructions to the actors to perform certain actions or behaviors—cry, laugh, look mad, walk over there, do a stunt, slam the door, and so forth.

The overall concept of genetics is like screenwriting, while epigenetics is like directing. The director puts his or her personal stamp on a film by choosing to omit or embellish certain scenes, actions, or dialogue, altering the movie for good or bad. After all, Alfred Hitchcock's finished film would be totally different than Stephen Spielberg's for the same movie script, right?

Like a director controls the film, you can control your epigenetics—and therefore, you can stop and reverse inflammation—as long as you understand the triggers and what to do about them. Here's a look at the major factors involved:

Obesity

This is a major cause of chronic inflammation. Fat cells release pro-inflammatory proteins called cytokines, which directly impact the lining of our arteries, leading to cardiovascular disease.

Researchers at the Free University in Amsterdam observed that overweight people definitely show symptoms of chronic, low-grade inflammation and were in danger of developing clogged arteries.

In collaboration with the National Institute on Aging in Bethesda, Maryland, the researchers analyzed health data on 16,600 adults in the US. These people had been followed between 1988 and 1994 as part of the third National Health and Nutrition Survey (NHANES III), a massive federal health study.

In their analysis, it was discovered that overweight people are far more likely than lean ones to have excess concentrations of C-reactive protein (CRP) in their blood. CRP is a gauge of inflammation because the body produces it while fighting infections. What's more, people showing even moderately elevated concentrations of CRP face a high risk of developing heart disease.

Measuring Inflammation

Your doctor has probably had your CRP levels measured as part of your annual blood work. But there are additional inflammation tests available. The Cleveland Heart Lab has developed an inflammatory blood panel that I use on most of my patients. It measures levels of the antioxidant CoQ10 and the oxidized form of LDL (Low Density Lipoprotein), a great determinant for arterial plaque formation.

This blood panel also measures ADMA (asymmetric dimethylarginine) and SDMA (symmetric dimethylarginine). These are substances that are found in your bloodstream when certain proteins are broken down. ADMA and SDMA interfere with the production of nitric oxide (NO), a molecule that helps dilate blood vessels and maintain a healthy endothelium (inner artery wall). Therefore, elevated levels of ADMA and SDMA may cause endothelial damage, increasing the risk of heart disease and stroke.

Finally, urine microalbumin is an early measure for endothelial inflammation. A measure called F2 isoprostane/microalbumin ratio tells if you are living a healthy lifestyle. Other excellent predictors for heart disease risk detected by this panel are LPLAC 2 and myeloperoxidase. Ask your physician about ordering this test, in addition to testing for CRP.

Lack of Exercise

A big promoter of obesity, a sedentary lifestyle causes inflammation of the arterial lining called the intima and thickens the inner wall (endothelium), triggering damage to the blood vessels. The small areas of damage to the intima essentially are like pimples inside the artery. When the pimple bursts, it releases macrophages to repair the intima.

Unfortunately, the cell environment allows deposits of fat and calcium to form, leading to hardening of the arteries, or *atherosclerosis*. The endpoint can be clot formation and a blocked artery. This can lead to the abrupt cessation of blood to part of the heart muscle and sudden death (called an acute myocardial infarction).

It might surprise you to know that often the only sign of heart disease is death from a clotted heart artery. Put another way: *The earliest sign of heart disease is death.*

I have always told my patients that you are lucky if you get chest pains—angina pectoris—or jaw pain or shortness of breath or fatigue. Why? Because the majority of patients' only warning sign is to die (not a very comforting symptom, I don't think).

This is why one of the lifestyle choices I always harp on is physical activity. Therefore, a lack of exercise is serious because of the cascade of inflammatory actions it initiates, which can lead to lethal heart disease.

High Glycemic Diets

These are diets loaded with foods and toxins that raise blood sugar. I'm talking about bread, rice, pasta, potatoes, sugar, and sweets—all of which not only create oxidation, but promote inflammation, too.

High-glycemic diets also elevate insulin levels, which inhibit our ability to burn fat. Insulin is by itself an inflammatory hormone (actually insulin was one of the first peptides discovered in humans). Although insulin is necessary, in excess amounts, it inflames the body.

Electromagnetic Fields (EMFs)

I can't believe that we slap warning labels on cigarettes and tobacco products regarding cancer, yet we continue to ignore something very serious and potentially lethal: the biological effects of radiation from electromagnetic fields (RE-EMFs). This is the radiofrequency by which all wireless technology operates, including not just cell towers and cell phones but Wi-Fi hubs and Wi-Fi-capable computers, "smart" utility meters, and even cordless home phones.

The World Health Organization (WHO) has concluded that cell phone use, specifically, is "possibly carcinogenic to humans," a rating that places mobiles in the middle of a rating scale that contains five levels of carcinogens. This means that cell phones are ranked just below things that are definitely known to cause cancer like smoking and tanning beds!

In Germany, researchers studied 1,000 residents who had lived near two cell phone towers for about ten years. During the last five years of the observations, researchers discovered neighbors living within 400 meters of the cell towers were diagnosed with cancer at a rate that was three times higher than those who lived much further away.

I'm not surprised. EMFs cause chronic inflammation in the body and have been linked to a wide range of diseases and disorders, including cancer, hormone dysfunction, and problems with the central nervous system, dementia, Parkinson's, anxiety, and depression. EMFs are also said to be a cause of a condition known as electrical sensitivity.

For perspective, EMFs disrupt cellular function throughout the body and interfere with sleep, hormone production, neurological function, immune response, and our ability to heal. EMFs also reduce our melatonin levels. Melatonin is an important anti-aging hormone that works as an antioxidant to protect cells from genetic damage that can lead to cancer, as well as neurological, cardiac, and reproductive damage.

EMFs also have been shown in research to trigger oxidative stress in cells—which, of course, accelerates aging and contributes to serious diseases.

I believe the problem with EMFs is going to get worse, with an even more widespread electronic-charged environment. The reason is that our cell towers are moving into a *5G network*, which is extremely high in radiation. The possible dangers to human health are headaches, infertility, aches and pain, and potential harm to bodily organs, including the skin, eyes, and heart, among other concerns.

The National Cancer Institute provides a handy chart to help you understand the levels of EMFs.

The Electromagnetic Spectrum

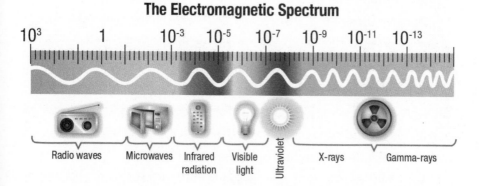

There are actions you can take to limit EMF exposure:

- Keep your cell phone and computer at a distance when possible.
- Unplug your Wi-Fi at night.
- Use your speakerphone rather than Bluetooth headsets.
- Stand as far away as possible from your microwave oven when heating food. It would be much better to avoid using the microwave for any reason.
- Keep your bedroom clear from as many electrical devices as possible, especially TVs and computers.
- Avoid installing low-voltage (12-volt) halogen, fluorescent tube, and energy-efficient cwaves (CFL).

Gut Issues

Starchy, sugary foods inflame the entire digestive tract, leading to many gastrointestinal ailments, including stomach and colon cancer, as well as destruction of friendly gut bacteria, collectively called the microbiome. Once bacteria are changed, unfriendly pathologic organisms can proliferate and cause various gastrointestinal problems, such as heartburn, irritable bowel syndrome, SIBO (small intestinal bacterial overgrowth), food allergies, and eventually, autoimmune disease (which were virtually unknown one hundred years ago). With autoimmune disease, antibodies attack otherwise healthy tissue.

To solve these conditions, many people reach for over-the-counter drugs or prescription medications. However, a simple symptom such as heartburn is made much worse when you take antacids or proton pump inhibitors like Prilosec or Prevacid. Such drugs lower the pH of the stomach and actually set you up for the digestive distress discussed above. With continued use of drugs, the power of the immune system eventually erodes and in fact promotes autoimmunity.

Autoimmune diseases begin to plague the body in various ways. One is leaky gut syndrome (also known as increased intestinal permeability)—a digestive condition in which harmful bacteria and toxins are able to "leak" through the intestinal wall. The digestion of food becomes incomplete, and the gut barrier has openings large enough for undigested particles to pass through, causing further immune reactions and inflammation. The harmful bacteria, thriving on sugar and grain, produce toxins, which now leak into the bloodstream.

A leaky gut gives rise to food sensitivities and allergies to peanuts, wheat, gluten, and dairy; the gut becomes irritable and cannot absorb even good foods. With autoimmune disease, there is chronic, body-wide inflammation—almost all lifestyle related and iatrogenic (caused by medical treatments). The gut must be repaired in order for this inflammation to stop. I'll discuss gut repair in the next chapter.

Believe it or not, this gut problem has a negative effect on the brain, which, like the gut, also has a barrier called the blood brain barrier (BBB). It protects the delicate brain cells from toxins in the blood. This barrier also has tight junctions that can get attacked by the same antibodies that attack the tight junctions in the gut. The result is that when you have a leaky gut, you are almost guaranteed to have a leaky brain as well.

Remember those toxins produced by the pathogenic bacteria in the gut that got into the blood? They will now get into the brain by that route as well and basically poison the brain. This mechanism has been linked to a lot of mental disorders as well as developmental problems like the autism spectrum. Many cases have been improved or even reversed by restoring gut function and bacterial flora.

Smoking

This stoppable habit creates a great deal of inflammation in our arteries and lung tissue, leading to increased incidence of heart attacks, strokes, emphysema, and lung cancer. In my entire career as a heart surgeon, I never operated on a woman for coronary artery disease who was not a smoker at some time in her life.

Cigarettes thicken the inner wall of all arteries called the endothelium. The thickening eventually leads to artery wall inflammation. The vessel itself undergoes wear and tear, caused by an abnormal buildup of platelets. Scar tissue is created as a result, and the scar tissue then calcifies into plaques. The vessel is either narrowed or a clot forms, and death can and does ensue. Inflammation is the chief culprit in all coronary artery disease.

Heavy Metal Toxicity

Exposure to metals such as mercury, lead, arsenic, and cadmium are becoming more prevalent as a cause of inflammation. These environmental toxins are rampant in our foods, including fish, as well as in products used in dentistry, MRIs, and x-rays. Not only do they trigger inflammation, they also destroy immune cells.

Sadly, most physicians don't realize that when patients complain of inflammation-related conditions, like joint pain, brain fog, memory loss, tremors, chronic fatigue, and headaches, that heavy metal toxicity is at the root of these issues. Becoming aware of, and addressing, these toxicities can save your life. You can be tested for heavy metal toxicity.

Stress

Chronic stress starts in the brain in response to fear, worry, and other negative emotions. But its influences on the body roam far and wide, working insidiously through the endocrine, neurological, and immune systems and endangering the heart, encouraging tumors, and tearing down bodily defenses against illnesses. It's not surprising that stress hurts our health; as George Bernard Shaw wrote over a century ago, "the sound body is a product of the sound mind."

Stress can cause chronic inflammation by producing changes in our hormones, and lowering our anti-inflammatory defenses. Cortisol, the stress hormone made in the adrenal glands, has many actions. Some of these actions protect us, but too much cortisol is destructive to tissues. It also damages the blood-brain barrier, which means pro-inflammatory substances can enter the brain and inflame it. Too much stress is the underlying cause of this form of inflammation.

Stress can also prompt gut inflammation and intestinal spasms, leading to more gastrointestinal (GI) symptoms, which can just translate to more stress or anxiety. It is a vicious cycle!

Suffice it to say that for now everything that you think you are exposed to in your internal and external environment can induce inflammation. It is now thought that this process is the universal cause of all disease; therefore, it is very important to understand in order to bring about a healing, youthful state.

ASK DR. BOB: How can I tell if I'm at risk for stroke?

A very simple noninvasive test is to measure the thickness of the carotid artery which goes up the neck to the brain. If its intimal thickness is greater than 1 millimeter at any age, you may be at serious risk.

4

Solution:

INFLAMMABOTS— THE NEW INFLAMMATION FIGHTERS

Some years ago, in line at Home Depot, I heard a voice behind me: "Dr. Willix?"

It was the wife of one of my patients, Phil, and her face was tight with worry. "We were just talking about you. I can't believe you're here," she said. "Phil needs to see you right away."

We stepped out of line, and her story tumbled out in a rush. "He wasn't sick, but he started having these odd issues with his memory. Then the seizures started, and his doctor ordered a CAT scan. They found a brain tumor. They can't operate because the tumor is too widespread. The oncologist says there's no treatment that can guarantee long-term survival and gave us little hope. Phil was planning to call you. He knows you've studied integrative and alternative medicine and wants to know what you think."

The very next day, I met with Phil. His diagnosis: glioblastoma mul-
tiforme, the same type of brain tumor that killed Senator Ted Kennedy
and Senator John McCain. You can imagine that these two senators
had access to the best that conventional medicine had to offer, yet their
prognosis was grim. Even with optimal conventional treatment, which
includes radiation therapy and chemotherapy, fewer than 10 percent of
people who have it survive five years. Phil's surgeon and oncologist had
already declared that he would die within the year.

Phil sought me out because he knew that I think outside the normal medical bag. I agreed to treat him. The deciding factor was his tre-
mendous will to live. This will, by the way, has a powerful effect on the
immune system. This fact, coupled with his strong faith as a minister,
gave me an exciting advantage. I've learned through the years of treating
cancer patients that spirituality, desire, and lack of fear are key factors
in positive long-term results and have a potent effect on natural killer
cells and the immune system.

You may have heard the term "psycho-neuro-endocrine-immunology."
This is one of the latest branches of scientific medicine. It shows us
that the mind and body are connected (which is what I call the Apollo
Factor, covered in the last chapter of this book). There is a great deal
of information that says that a positive attitude (thoughts = psycho)
sends a signal to the CNS (central nervous system = neuro) that in turn
creates a chemical hormone (endocrine), and it stimulates the action
of various immune cells. Phil's combined belief in God and his strong
desire to live to see his children become adults ignited an energetic and
anti-inflammatory response to heal the physical body.

I met with Phil, convinced that he would do anything to get well,
including opening his mind to a belief system and therapies I use with
my patients every day. He believed that if he was meant to heal, it would
be for a higher calling or purpose for his future.

From that point on, Phil's surgeon and oncologist simply monitored his condition, ready to prescribe medications if necessary, and acted only as observers—skeptical observers at that! They had made their diagnosis and waited for it to play out. In other words, they did not believe he could or would survive, so they offered no hope. Nor did they offer any solutions to comfort Phil, his wife, and his children.

My faith, however, rests in the world of possibilities. Possibilities lie in the field of quantum mechanics—the belief that what you focus on, you create—and the field of epigenetics—the ways in which environmental factors, such as nutrition, pollution, emotional stress, physical trauma, and other factors—can affect our DNA and genetic blueprint, good or bad. I put my money and Phil's on infinite possibilities, and he agreed.

To Phil and his wife, my treatment must have seemed absurdly basic. First, I put Phil on a plant-based diet—no animal protein and no simple sugars. All cancers can be fed by sugar and high-glycemic carbohydrates, but all of the cancer-fighting antioxidants and anti-inflammatory foods come from plants. Fruits have benefit only if they are high in nutritional compounds called carotenoids and flavonoids. My forty-plus years of study on nutrition have led me to become even stricter about the value of nutritional elements and healing DNA and the mitochondria. I want to limit further DNA mutation, as well as quench inflammation and feed the immune macrophages what they need to protect the cells.

Because I am trained in Ayurveda (translated it means the "knowledge of life"), one of the oldest systems of natural medicine in the world, I "prescribed" Ayurvedic herbal remedies because of their combined antioxidant and anti-inflammatory medicinal value but few, if any, side effects. I also taught Phil several types of meditation, including *centering prayer* and visualization to heal from his tumor. He practiced these techniques twice daily for twenty to thirty minutes each session. During the day, he concentrated on informing his tumor that he had no use for it anymore, it had served its purpose, and now it was no longer needed.

Phil followed my therapies to the letter. In a few weeks, the frequency and severity of his seizures began to lessen. His memory cleared, and he began to feel healthy again. He took my nutritional program to the next level and began not only a vegan plan but a raw-food vegan program. His follow-up CT scans showed no progression of the tumor at six months. Miraculously, the scans began to show a regression of the tumor after one year.

Seven years and several MRIs later, there was no evidence of his tumor! It had vanished, along with his memory problems.

The last I heard, Phil was teaching others with cancer a nutritional plan to reduce the progression of their disease. His neurosurgeon certainly couldn't teach them. In fact, the surgeon conceded that he'd never seen a recovery like Phil's—something special had been at work.

Indeed there had been. Phil had activated his epigenes and applied the Apollo Factor (see chapter 16) to change his DNA messengers and increase his immune cells. This boosted the body's innate intelligence to heal itself—and did so without drugs. His nutrition decreased the inflammation, and the herbs helped raise his immunity. In short, Phil made life-saving epigenetic changes through diet, meditation, and imagery. All of these actions, working synergistically, resulted in a miraculous outcome.

Clearly, there's plenty you can do to tame and even prevent such simmering inflammation from provoking and exacerbating ill health, even death, and forestalling age-related diseases. I will cover meditation in chapter 14, but there are several key actions you can take now to fight inflammation in your body.

Harness the Power of Inflammabots

What exactly is an "inflammabot"?

If you went to the dictionary and looked up the word *inflammabot*, you wouldn't find it. That is because I made the word up. But it is an apt new word because it best describes any substance or chemical or body signal that stops or slows down inflammation. Examples of inflammabots include certain foods, good fats, herbs, and enzymes, to name a just a few items. Here is a closer look.

Anti-Aging Fats

Plant-sourced oils are major inflammabots. My favorites for anti-aging are the following:

Coconut oil. This fat is high in fatty components called medium chain triglycerides (MCTs). Due to their shorter length, MCTs are easily digested and possess many health benefits. One is that MCTs can even significantly reduce C-reactive protein (CRP), the inflammatory marker that increases the risk of heart disease.

Coconut oil and its MCTs also help fight overweight and obesity, which cause inflammation. MCTs can increase how many calories you burn compared to the same number of calories from longer chain fats. They also rev up your metabolism, which stimulates fat burning.

There is evidence that cultures that have eaten coconuts as a staple in their diets have a very low incidence of heart disease and tend to be very healthy in general.

One healthy habit is to get a fresh coconut when it is available. Drink the coconut water and then eat the coconut meat over the next few days. Or you can use coconut oil as a salad dressing or condiment over vegetables. You can also bake with it.

Olive oil. Although it does contain saturated fats, the predominant fatty acid in olive oil is a monounsaturated fat called oleic acid. Studies suggest that oleic acid reduces inflammation and may even have beneficial effects in switching off genes linked to cancer.

Evidence from Mediterranean cultures, where olive oil is the chief fat, has convinced me that this oil has strong inflammabot qualities. Case in point: The Prevención con Dieta Mediterránea (PREDIMED) study is the largest trial investigating the potential cardiovascular protective effects of the olive-oil rich Mediterranean diet. The study involved 7,172 Spanish patients with a high risk of suffering from a cardiovascular-related event. These patients were randomized into three different diets: a Mediterranean diet supplemented with extra-virgin olive oil, a Mediterranean diet supplemented with mixed nuts, and a low-fat control diet.

Initial analysis of the study found that, after approximately five years, those on the olive-oil supplemented Mediterranean diet had a 37 percent lower relative risk of all-cause mortality when compared to those on the other diets. Further, in-depth analysis on a subset of 200 high-risk patients found that those on the Mediterranean diet had reduced blood pressure after one year, compared to those on the control diet. Other studies suggest that if this were the only source of monounsaturated fat you eat, you'll live longer and avoid strokes.

It is easy to use olive oil in your daily diet to harness similar benefits. Monounsaturated fats are also quite resistant to high heat, making extra-virgin olive oil a healthy choice for cooking. Use it on salads and in cooking daily, if you choose. Its benefits far out way the amount of fat that it will bring into your diet.

Avocado. I love avocadoes. The Aztecs considered them important for sexual vigor. If that's true, I'm all in. Many people ask me whether they contain too much fat. The percentage of fat is really not important because it contains the desirable and protective fat—the monounsaturated kind. Avocadoes are packed with B vitamins and monounsaturated fat.

Both the avocado and avocado oil have been found to protect against prostate and breast cancer, as well as help treat arthritis. They also help prevent heart disease and high blood pressure. The antioxidant lutein in avocado protects your eyes. Avocado oil brings back a youthful-looking skin.

When your children have a burn or cut, the oil can act as a healing balm on the wound. Also, try using avocado oil on your psoriasis or contact dermatitis rather than harsh pharmacological remedies used by many conventional doctors.

I eat avocadoes any time of the day, even at breakfast when I like to combine them with tomatoes and spinach or kale. Of course, I love guacamole for snacking and on Mexican food, along with two other inflammabots: jalapenos and garlic.

Clary Sage Oil. One of the healing pearls in nature is the clary sage plant. Mentioned in the Old Testament of the Bible (the Torah), it was named "the eye of God" for its unique beauty.

Clary sage oil is high in an essential omega-3 fat called alpha-linolenic acid (ALA). Clary sage and ALA can actually help the brain work better because the oil is capable of crossing the blood-brain barrier, improving the function of the cells and protecting the mitochondria.

High levels of ALA are more anti-inflammatory than omega-3 fats from fish. ALA also improves your immune system. Two tablespoons of clary sage oil or three to six capsules daily will give you all the inflammabot protection you need.

Seeds and Nuts. Foods such as chia seeds, pomegranate seeds, almonds, and other nuts should be a regular part of your diet. They are high in anti-inflammatory fats.

But avoid peanuts (which are technically legumes, not nuts). They often contain toxic mold. The same advice goes for peanut butter because it is typically high in sugar. Other nut and seed butters, such as almond, sunflower, and cashew butters are healthier choices.

Further, nut milks are an excellent way to access anti-inflammatory benefits. I recommend almond, hazelnut, walnut, and soy milks instead of cow's milk, which promotes inflammation.

Flavonoids

These are compounds found in fruits, vegetables, teas, and cocoa. They have been called "nature's biologic modifiers" because they have the ability to modify the body's reaction to compounds such as allergens, viruses, and substances that cause cancer.

Flavonoids have received substantial interest because of their antioxidant properties together with the ability to inhibit the secretion of pro-inflammatory substances. Research shows that a flavonoid-rich diet improves blood flow, thus reducing the risk of cardiovascular disease.

In general, flavonoids fight free radicals, carcinogens, and aging in general. Some help normalize blood sugar and iron out wrinkles by promoting healthy collagen in your skin.

The most powerful action of these inflammabots, however, is found in the realm of epigenetics. They can help turn off the genes that make aging happen.

Some common sources of flavonoids include:

Blueberries

Strawberries

Red apples with the skin

Red grapes

Cherries

Black tea

Onions and scallions

Broccoli

Kale

Spinach

Parsley

Thyme

Hot peppers

Citrus fruits, including grapefruit, oranges, and lemons

Soybeans and other legumes

To get more flavonoids in your body, think in terms of food colors. The more colorful the fruits and vegetables are on your plate, the more flavonoids you're eating. Eat a variety of colors, too—greens, reds, purples, blues, yellows, and oranges.

Water and Hydration

It is fascinating to me that most people do not know that water is the most important nutrient in the human body. More than 80 percent of our body is made up of water, and yet we rarely think of it as a nutrient.

Drinking ample water is one of the easiest ways to douse inflammation because it halts inflammation in tissues, such as cartilage. Your joints then operate well and move with all the fluidity of youth. So in that sense, water is definitely an inflammabot.

I am often asked, "What type of water should I drink?"

Well, that is a question even I struggle with at times. My gut reaction is "rain water" because it contains minerals. But it might pick up toxins from poor air quality, so you'd have to consider how good the air quality is in your particular area.

If I lived in a pristine, remote area of the world, I would drink from mountain streams. I used to go wilderness camping on my motorcycle into the provincial parks of Ontario and Quebec, where I'd drink from streams. These days, though, they are contaminated from agricultural run-off, pesticides, and possibly sewage sludge.

I'm sure most people don't want to collect rain water or drink from streams, anyway! The next best thing is to make sure your water is filtered, so you get rid of the bromides and chlorines from the tap.

Alkalinized water with a pH of 8.0 or greater is a good choice, too. I'm not a fan of distilled water because it contains no minerals and therefore is not alkalinizing.

Don't drink from plastic glasses or containers or bottles; they contain toxins that leach into the water.

As far as how much to drink, I believe aiming for six to eight 8-ounce glasses daily is a reasonable target.

Natural Enzymes

Many people aren't aware of what enzymes do or why they are so critical to our existence. Think of enzymes as little "spark plugs." Produced by all living things, they are catalysts that either initiate chemical reactions or speed up chemical reactions already in progress.

We need enzymes for everything that goes on in the body, including digestion, breathing, and circulation. Enzymes also attack disease, fight inflammation, and slow down the aging process. In fact, the power to do all of this is directly related to how strong and well-populated your body is with your enzymes.

Foods are such rich sources of enzymes. These include pineapple (the source of the enzyme *bromelain)* and papaya (the source *of papain).* Any raw, fresh fruit or vegetable is a powerful enzyme source, but only if the enzymes have not been destroyed by heat—which is why I advocate eating raw foods.

Ayurveda, Aging, and Inflammation

I have long practiced Ayurveda, one of the world's most authoritative mind-body-spirit medicinal systems. This system of medicine includes therapies for healthy aging so as to create optimal health and longevity. Almost two hundred Ayurvedic plants and herbs have been identified that exhibit anti-inflammatory activities. Here is a rundown of several of the most well-known anti-inflammatory agents used for centuries to treat aging and chronic diseases.

Garlic extract (Allium Sativum). This agent has been used to reduce inflammation in irritable bowel syndrome, help prevent arteries from clogging, and treat arthritis and other inflammatory conditions.

Aloe vera. The gel from the leaves of this plant has long been used in the treatment of a variety of disorders including wounds and burns. In addition to its wound-healing benefit, aloe vera has antidiabetic and hypoglycemic properties. It also contains an active component called emodin that exerts anti-inflammatory and anti-cancer effects.

Bacopa monnieri. Extracts from this plant have been reported to significantly improve short-term and long-term memory.

Boswellia serrata. Extracts from this Indian Ayurvedic medicinal plant have been used for centuries in traditional Ayurvedic medicine for a wide variety of inflammatory diseases, including inflammatory bowel disease. It has been shown to help halt the growth of many tumor cells, including glioma, colon cancer, leukemia cells, human melanoma, and prostate cancer cells.

Chicory (Cichorium intybus). Chicory roots have been used as a digestive aid, diuretic, laxative, and mild sedative, as well as possessing anti-inflammatory and liver-protecting benefits.

Cinnamon (Cinnamomum cassia). This popular spice is used to cure various inflammation-related diseases such as rheumatism, sprains, bronchitis, and muscle pains. It also has antimicrobial, laxative, analgesic (pain-killing), diuretic, and antidiabetic activity.

Guggul. This is a plant compound derived from the gum resin of the tree *Commiphora mukul* grown in India. This resin has been employed in Ayurvedic medicine for centuries to treat obesity, bone fractures, arthritis, inflammation, and heart disease. It is available in supplement form.

Garcinia cambogia. This is an edible fruit native to southeastern Asia. The rind is often brewed into a tea to help alleviate joint inflammation and bowel irregularities. The fruit's active ingredient is hydroxycitric acid (HCA), which helps curb appetite and cravings, blocks the body's production of fat, and boosts energy.

Ginger (Zingiber officinale). Ginger has long been used to treat a wide range of conditions, including stomachaches, nausea, vomiting, headaches, and arthritis. Ginger is rich in substances called gingerols and shogaols that have antioxidant, anti-inflammatory, and anticarcinogenic properties. A number of recent studies have renewed interest in ginger for the treatment of chronic inflammatory conditions.

Licorice (Glycyrrhiza glabra). Here is a medicinal plant whose dried roots and stolons form an important component of various Ayurvedic formulations. Licorice is reported to have anti-inflammatory, anticancer, antimicrobial, antioxidant, and liver-protective benefits. Other than these, licorice extract also has antidepressant properties.

Piper nigrum. You know this better as black pepper, but it is a medicine, a preservative, and a perfume in many Asian countries. An extract of the active phenolic component, piperine, it stimulates the digestive enzymes of the pancreas, protects against oxidative cell damage, and acts as an anti-inflammatory.

Turmeric (Curcuma longa). I discussed this spice in chapter 2. It deserves additional mention here because of its long history of use in Ayurvedic medicine as a treatment for inflammatory conditions.

Probiotics and Prebiotics

Aging is related to changes in your gut microbiome, which is made up of more than 100 trillion organisms. As you get older, the bacterial population in your gut gradually shifts toward a disease-promoting, rather than a disease-preventing, state simply as a result of the aging process. The gut microbiome can also be destroyed by certain drugs, including statins, antibiotics, and protein pump inhibitors. Also, the gut is very susceptible to inflammation, which harms healthy gut bacteria.

In the early 1900s, a Russian zoologist named Elie Metchnikoff reported that Bulgarian peasants who consumed large quantities of fermented milk, such as yogurt, lived long lives. He attributed their longevity to the health-promoting effects of the live microorganisms (probiotics) in the milk. Probiotics are live bacteria with many health benefits. They are found in fresh fermented products, such as yogurt, but not if they are found on the shelf. The number of live organisms

Probiotics Strengthen Your Natural Defenses

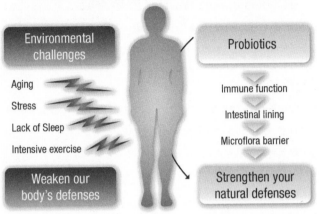

in store-bought fermented milk products is diminished or nonexistent once it is more than a few hours to a day old. So please do not tell me you are eating yogurt for the probiotics. The studies on longevity are written about populations that are making the products fresh—not refrigerated.

Thanks to his early work, we know today that you can slow aging down by taking probiotic supplements. They have been shown to reduce markers of age-related inflammation and organ damage. Probiotics have been well studied in human trials and animal models. For example, a statistical analysis of fifteen studies with 788 subjects showed effective lowering of cardiovascular risk factors, such as total cholesterol, LDL cholesterol, and inflammatory markers, with probiotic supplementation. I recommend taking 50–100 billion colonies of a probiotic supplement daily.

There are other moves you can take to promote healthy gut flora. One is to include *prebiotic* foods in your diet. These are nondigestible carbohydrates that act as food for probiotics and help them thrive. Using probiotics and eating prebiotics food is called *symbiotic* and is a relevant anti-aging strategy.

Most prebiotics are complex carbohydrates present in whole grains, fruits and vegetables, or are produced industrially. My picks for the top fifteen prebiotic foods are the following; please note that they are all plant-based:

Chicory root
Dandelion greens (as long as the lawn has not been treated with
    dangerous herbicides or pesticides)
Jerusalem artichoke
Garlic
Onions
Leeks
Asparagus
Bananas
Barley
Oats
Apple
Flaxseeds
Jicama
Seaweed
Cocoa

Watch Out for Endotoxins!

As a normal part of their life cycle, bacteria will die off. When certain types of bacteria die, they give off components that are toxic. Specifically, they release lipopolysaccharides (LPS). LPS are natural components of some bacteria membranes (even healthy ones).

As long as your gut is healthy, your body can handle this process without incident. But if your gut is unhealthy or leaky, LPS slips into the bloodstream and triggers inflammation throughout the body. This state is called endotoxemia, and it can be highly destructive to your health.

LPS-induced endotoxemia is linked to:

Aging

Weight gain

Chronic constipation

Mood disorders such as depression and anxiety

Memory problems

Chronic pain

Parkinson's disease and Alzheimer's disease

Low testosterone

Insulin resistance

Atherosclerosis

Autoimmune disease

Naturally, you want to prevent endotoxemia at all costs. One of the most important actions you can take is in the area of diet. Avoid high-fat and processed foods, especially, because they irritate the gut.

In fact, research shows that just one single processed, high-fat and high-carbohydrate meal can increase the level of LPS in our bloodstream many-fold. LPS can remain elevated in the bloodstream over the course of weeks and months.

Case in point: An important study, published in *Diabetes Care* in 2009, found that a 900-calorie "American Heart Association" (AHA) meal of oatmeal, milk, orange juice, raisins, peanut butter, and English muffin prevented post-meal endotoxemia, whereas a meal of egg and sausage muffin sandwiches with hash browns did not. The former meal, which was largely plant-based with the exception of milk, also prevented rise in various markers of oxidative stress.

Other preventive actions include:

- Reducing emotional stress in your life. Stress increases inflammation, which increases endotoxin absorption.
- Taking probiotic supplements regularly because they heal the gut and keep it healthy.
- Including coconut oil in your diet. Coconut helps inhibit bacterial endotoxin growth while at the same time healing the intestines.

- Eating prebiotic foods. The indigestible fibers found in these foods prevent the absorption of endotoxins in the intestine and can reduce the production of stress hormones that worsen endotoxin contamination.

Lifestyle Inflammabots

The way you live your life can influence the healing power of inflammabots—or not. Certain lifestyle choices will halt inflammation-related aging:

- Maintain an ideal body weight with a low body fat percentage (14–20 percent in men and 18–22 percent in women).
- Don't smoke.
- Don't drink too much alcohol (keep consumption to less than six ounces of liquor or thirty ounces of wine per week).
- Exercise regularly with HIIT (High Intensity Interval Training) for your heart, weight training to prevent muscle loss, and yoga or Tai Qi for flexibility. (See chapter 10 for more information on physical activity.)
- Get six to ten hours of sleep per night.
- Keep up with good oral hygiene to avoid gum disease, which can spread inflammation throughout your body.

The more I study the mechanism of inflammation, the more I see that the body can repair and rejuvenate itself—as long as you give it the right resources. Food, supplements, enzymes, and lifestyle choices are vital strategies for stopping inflammation-related aging and staying youthful.

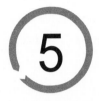

5

DECLINING HORMONES AND PEPTIDES

If you want to trade your body in for a new model, you've got to address the third significant cause of aging: dwindling hormones and peptides. Our bodies are programmed to start declining after about the age of twenty-one. That's when we see hormones start to decline and peptides begin to weaken. However, we can *pick up* the activity of these important hormones and peptides.

What Are Hormones?

The word *hormone* comes from the Greek, meaning "stir up." Hormones are responsible for numerous bodily processes, including growth, metabolism, and sexual function. They dictate body temperature and weight, and orchestrate the body's response during moments of stress.

Think of hormones like keys: without a companion lock, the key won't work. But once the hormone key fits the right cellular lock (the "receptor"), the cell opens up and a response is triggered. I'll use the example of human growth hormone (HGH); this response can be muscle or bone growth, or cellular repair.

But once we get to an age in which further growth and fertility are behind us, we simply don't produce as many hormones. Those we do produce get dispatched with reduced frequency. Like a worn-out lock, receptors also become less sensitive as we age, so even if the hormones are sent, sometimes their keys no longer work. When this occurs body-wide—hormone keys failing to unlatch trillions of cellular locks—the signs of aging start appearing.

Hormones are produced by our endocrine system; this includes the hypothalamus, pituitary, thyroid, adrenals, parathyroids, sexual organs (ovaries and testes), and pancreas.

Of these sites, the hypothalamus, pituitary, and the adrenal glands deserve special mention. The hypothalamus and pituitary glands are located just above the brainstem, while the adrenal glands are found on top of the kidneys. The hypothalamus tells the pituitary gland to stimulate the thyroid, sex organs, parathyroid, and adrenals to make the blood-borne endocrine hormones.

The hypothalamus, pituitary, and adrenal glands make up the hypothalamic-pituitary-adrenal (HPA) axis. It forms a network that loops between your nervous system and your stress hormones. When you're up against a big stressful situation, your hypothalamus churns out a hormone called CRH. It signals your pituitary gland to discharge another hormone—ACTH—into your bloodstream. That hormone, in turn, tells your adrenal glands to release the stress hormones cortisol and adrenaline.

All of this works well for a while (the faster heart rate and blood pressure from all that adrenaline help you flee from any stressor or predator), but if the stress doesn't stop, these chemicals stay high and turn against you, compromising your immune system, exhausting your adrenal glands, throwing your cholesterol levels out of whack, and ultimately causing you to age faster than you should. Dysfunction of the HPA axis may also contribute to aging-related diseases like depression, loss of muscle mass, cognitive deficits, and Alzheimer's disease in some older individuals.

Several events can cause dysfunction of the HPA. One is head trauma, commonly seen in prize fighters, football players, and victims of automobile accidents. Others are oxidative stress and telomere shortening.

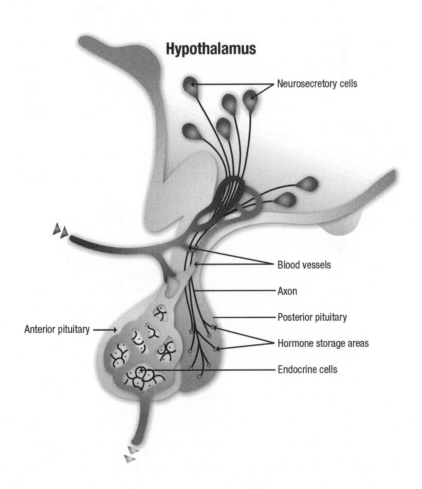

Hypothalamus

Neurosecretory cells

Blood vessels

Axon

Posterior pituitary

Anterior pituitary

Hormone storage areas

Endocrine cells

The Anti-Aging Hormones

The major hormones associated with the aging process are: thyroid (TSH, T4, and T3), DHEA, cortisol, testosterone, estrogen, insulin, human growth hormone (HGH), and melatonin. Here's a brief look at how each of these works:

Thyroid Hormones

Thyroid hormones control metabolism, mood, weight, and temperature. An overactive thyroid causes anxiety, agitation, and weight loss, while an underactive thyroid triggers weight gain, depression, and thinning hair.

There are two major forms, T4 (thyroxin), which isn't as potent as the activated form, T3 (triiodothyronine). T4 is normally converted to the activated form of T3. T3 enhances energy, allowing a rapid response to a stress. People who are under chronic stress tend to overutilize their thyroid hormone and many of these people can end up having hypothyroidism, or low thyroid.

Thyroid disease is much more common in women than men, especially in the conversion of T4 to T3, creating the so-called ambulatory T3 syndrome. It is caused by inflammation, a leaky gut, an imbalanced microbiome (too many unfriendly bacteria), and a decline in estrogen as a woman ages. This syndrome is rarely recognized by most physicians.

You may have heard of TSH. It stands for "thyroid-stimulating hormone" and is produced by the pituitary gland in your brain. This gland tells your thyroid to make and release the thyroid hormones into your blood.

DHEA (Dehydroepiandrosterone)

Dehydroepiandrosterone, or DHEA, is produced by glands perched atop the kidneys, the adrenals. DHEA is the building block of two other anti-aging hormones: estrogen and testosterone. DHEA is most abundant in your body around age twenty-five; after that, production wanes and drops off dramatically by age sixty-five.

DHEA is believed to slow aging, increase bone and muscle strength, burn fat, boost immunity, and protect against many chronic diseases. Cosmetically, DHEA also increases the production of collagen, making skin appear smoother and younger looking. There has been considerable interest in using DHEA as a brain agent to treat Alzheimer's disease.

Aging Pioneers: John R. Lee, MD, and Daniel Rudman, MD

John R. Lee, MD, was an international authority and pioneer in the use of natural progesterone cream and natural hormone balance. His work in the 1980s opened the door for more people to talk about hormones and their effect on aging—in both women and men. Lee was the first to publish startling conclusions about conventional hormone replacement therapy (HRT from mare's urine) that it did not work as predicted and, worse, posed health threats to women. His findings ignited a firestorm of controversy. But newer research vindicated him and proved him right. Now millions of women who want to stay youthful are searching for alternatives to HRT and finding them in bioidentical hormones.

Lee showed physicians that using a plant extract, which resembled natural progesterone was safe and could stop the progression of osteoporosis and osteopenia (bone loss). This development led to the compounding of natural estrogens, including estradiol, the body's strongest and most prevalent female estrogen. From there, bioidentical progesterone, other estrogens, and even testosterone were compounded, giving physicians and their patients—both men and women—a significant anti-aging edge.

Despite the availability and effectiveness of these natural, bioidentical hormones, many physicians ignore them and use synthetic horse urine instead (Premarin). This tells me a lot about their credibility.

The final piece of the bioidentical hormone puzzle fell into place in 1990 with the work of Dr. Daniel Rudman, an endocrinologist and nutritionist, who devoted his research to the well-being of the frail and elderly.

He was the principal author of a paper in *The New England Journal of Medicine*, "Effect of human growth hormone in men over 60 years old." The study was based on a clinical trial of twenty-one healthy men, aged sixty-one to eighty-one. It found that after six months of injections of a genetically engineered version of the natural human growth hormone, the men emerged with bodies that by many measures were almost twenty years younger than the ones they started with. Thus began the anti-aging movement as it relates to hormonal replacement.

Let me state from the outset that in the last thirty-eight years, I have used bioidentical hormones to preserve health and prevent aging in thousands of patients safely and effectively.

This field of medicine is evolving all the time, but bioidentical hormones are here to stay. Now we have expanded our knowledge and have uncovered an even more exciting approach to aging by using the body's own natural signals for healing.

Cortisol

When faced with stress, your body naturally pumps out cortisol to help you deal with it. In small amounts, this hormone can provide the body with the necessary tools to escape a stressful situation. But if you suffer from chronically elevated cortisol, cortisol stays high even after the stress has ended. (So does adrenaline production.)

When there is the constant production of high levels of cortisol and adrenaline and nothing else, your body begins to break down, and premature aging can set in. You're more prone to illness and disease because your immune system is not working up to par.

Testosterone

Testosterone helps build muscle, burn fat, strengthen bones, and boost libido. In men, it also helps make sperm. Men produce testosterone in their testes. Women, who have much lower levels, make the hormone in their ovaries and adrenal glands.

For men and women, adequate levels of testosterone are associated with energy, enthusiasm, and improvements in mood, physical strength, muscle function, circulation, the immune system, and just about every other system in our body. With age, women tend to experience an increase in testosterone and a decline in estrogen, while men tend to experience the opposite—an increase in estrogen and a decline in testosterone.

Low testosterone increases a man's risk of heart disease, prostate cancer, and Alzheimer's disease.

Estrogen

Estrogen is commonly thought of as a sex hormone strictly involved in reproduction, but it has many other jobs in the body. Estrogen helps keep the skin smooth and moist and lubricates vaginal tissues. It also boosts high-density cholesterol (good cholesterol), and lowers low-density cholesterol (bad cholesterol), thus cutting the odds of developing heart disease. Estrogen is required for proper bone formation, particularly in women. When estrogen levels drop, women are at greater risk for elevated cholesterol, osteoporosis, and cardiovascular disease.

Progesterone

Produced by the ovaries, progesterone is referred to as the "pregnancy hormone" because it helps a woman's body achieve and maintain pregnancy. Progesterone levels fall during menopause as well as with chronic stress. Low levels are linked to premenstrual syndrome (PMS), fibrocystic breast disease, infertility, increased risk and incidence of miscarriage, as well as polycystic ovarian syndrome (PCOS). Men with prostate problems also tend to have low levels.

Insulin

Manufactured in the pancreas, insulin is a hormone that helps your cells use sugar (glucose) from the carbohydrates you eat for energy or to store glucose for later use. Insulin helps stabilize your blood sugar levels.

When cells become less sensitive to insulin, they don't readily accept glucose as well. Called insulin resistance, this situation often happens as we age and gain weight. The body then must crank out more insulin to keep glucose levels under control to avoid type 2 diabetes.

High levels of insulin can accelerate overall aging. This occurs when you eat too many foods high in sugar, such as pastries, muffins, candy, white pasta, white rice, and fruit juice—all of which spike blood sugar and insulin. Insulin is also a "peptide." (See page 105.)

HCG (Human Chorionic Gonadotropin)

HCG, also known as the pregnancy hormone, can be used to stimulate the production of testosterone in men and preserve atrophy of the testicles. It's also used for weight loss with a severe calorie-restricted diet.

Pregnenolone

Pregnenolone is used for fatigue and increasing energy; Alzheimer's disease and enhancing memory; as well as reducing stress and improving immunity.

Human Growth Hormone (HGH)

HGH is secreted by the pituitary gland located at the base of the brain. As its name implies, HGH regulates normal growth and development.

HGH is also known as the "youth hormone" because it protects your heart, lowers your body fat, increases muscle mass, boosts energy, and prevents aging. It is also essential for skin-cell repair and the prevention of sagging. It is used medically in the elderly to help tissue repair when immunity is compromised. It is also given to HIV-positive patients and after surgical procedures to accelerate the natural healing of tissues.

Supposedly, HGH declines at the rate of 15 percent per decade after the age of thirty. New research suggests, however, that the amount of HGH in the pituitary gland of a twenty-year-old and a hundred-year-old are the same. If HGH is in full supply in your system, why do levels decline? The reason is that it just doesn't release as well as it does when you're younger. The production of growth hormone is linked to our habits. If we don't exercise, sleep poorly, or do not eat enough protein, HGH will decline.

Melatonin

Frequent travelers and jet lag sufferers swear by melatonin supplements. Produced naturally by the pineal gland within the brain, melatonin regulates our sleep cycle, ramping up at night time and dropping off by morning. As an anti-aging hormone, it helps improve sleep and fights against free radicals that damage cells.

Menopause and Andropause

Although everyone recognizes that women go through the change of life called menopause, it has taken many decades for doctors to recognize that males go through hormonal changes as well. This change is called "andropause" or "manopause."

In women, it's fairly easy to recognize menopause because of irregular periods, hot flashes, weight gain, and other signs. But in men, the signs are more subtle.

As andropause kicks in, there is a decline in the pituitary hormone, luteinizing hormone, which normally stimulates the testicle to make more testosterone. So testosterone falls off without much warning. This typically triggers weight gain in a man—which is a clue that he might be going through andropause.

There is also decline in HGH and DHEA, all of which has a profound effect on a man's health, from muscle loss to increased risk of heart disease to premature aging. Fortunately, with testing and hormone supplementation, andropause can be managed and youthful vigor can be restored.

The New Science of Peptides and Aging

Besides hormones, other hormone-related proteins that influence aging are peptides—short chains of amino acids that help regulate cellular activity. The body's naturally occurring amounts of peptides decrease with age. Exciting new findings reveal that peptides promote self-healing at the level of the mitochondria (the energy factory of cells) and therefore can help reverse aging and help maintain your health as you get older.

Certain peptides can improve immune function, repair DNA, promote mitochondria function, boost memory, reduce anxiety and depression, prevent gut diseases, and repair ligaments and tendons. Others reverse some of the symptoms of Alzheimer's disease and decrease amyloid, the protein that damages the nerves of the brain.

Currently, a combination of bioidentical hormones with peptides is offering new strategies and promises in the field of anti-aging medicine.

Here is a summary of the most important anti-aging peptides and how they work:

Growth-Hormone Releasing Peptides

One of the most important is ghrelin, which is produced by the stomach. It is a potent stimulator of HGH release to help the body retain its youthfulness and exert an age-protecting effect. So rather than inject the body with HGH (the common route of administration), we can increase this hormone by using ghrelin-like peptides. This is a much safer approach.

Other growth-hormone-releasing peptides include sermorelin, tesamorelin, and CJC 1295. They signal the cells to release the growth hormone and do this through the hypothalamus.

BPC 157 (Body Protection Compound)

This peptide works by signaling the body to promote healing and decrease chronic inflammation. It can help treat autoimmune diseases, irritable bowel syndrome, Crohn's disease, and athletic injuries, like tendon and muscle tears. Further, it heals certain types of liver damage.

BPC 157 also:

- can protect the brain in post-traumatic stress and concussions;
- may help repair the blood gut brain axis;
- increases telomerase (te-LAW-mer-ace) and protects telomere shortening (See chapters 7 and 8);
- promotes healing and decreases chronic inflammation naturally;
- helps ease acid reflux and esophagitis;
- can relieve many of the autoimmune diseases of the bowel, including irritable bowel syndrome (IBS), Crohn's disease, and diverticulosis;
- repairs injuries from tendons and muscle tears.

The Healing Power of BPC 157

My son, an avid cyclist, triathlete, and Ultraman competitor, recently went to the Duke Sports Medicine Clinic to be treated for a stress fracture. He asked the doctors about BPC 157, but they had no idea what he was talking about, even though there has been extensive research on this compound.

So why aren't doctors well-versed in this peptide and others? The reason is simple: Peptides are natural products, many of which cannot be patented for specific use. That means that the pharmaceutical industry cannot control it. Duke Sports Medicine physicians and other doctors get their drug information largely from the pharmaceutical companies.

As for my son's injury, the standard treatment for his stress fracture is typically six weeks of rest—which for an active guy like my son—is always depressing. So he and I took a different approach. I used 0.1 cc (cubic centimeters) of BPC 157 injected in the area of his stress fracture of his foot, and within two weeks he was able to put enough pressure on it to walk and cycle, and eventually, he resumed his running so that he could compete in his next ultra-distance event.

Healing occurs because the peptide signals the body to repair. Years ago, I was excited about the value of stem cells. Now I know that the peptides can have an effect on stem cells and repair of almost any organ of human body. This is why peptides are such an exciting and profound area of medicine.

Thymosin Alpha 1 and Thymosin Beta 4 (TB4)

These peptides are beneficial in reducing inflammation. They are found in the thymus gland, where immune cells known as T cells mature and are released when prompted to do so.

Thymosin-alpha 1 (TA1):

- Is responsible for restoring immune functions;
- Is used in phase 3 clinical trials for the treatment of hepatitis C and phase 2 trials for hepatitis B;
- May eradicate unhealthy cells and stop an infection or cancer growth;
- Exhibits antibacterial and antifungal properties;
- Suppresses tumor growth;
- Protects against oxidative damage.

Thymosin-beta 4 (TB4):

This hormone is secreted by the thymus gland. Its primary purpose is to stimulate the production of T cells, important in the immune system. It:

- Plays a role in tissue repair;
- Is currently being evaluated as a potential therapy for HIV, AIDS, and influenza;
- Promotes normal cell function and survival;
- Is involved in the formation of blood vessels;
- Assists stem cells in maturing;
- Promotes the production of inflammation-fighting chemicals in the body.

RG3 (Synapsin)

This peptide, derived from ginseng, is an adaptogen, and when combined with NR (Nucleotide Riboside) and B12, as a nasal spray, it improves memory and brain function by depleting inflammatory brain factors called cytokines. It may reduce the amyloid plaque in Alzheimer's disease.

DSIP (Deep Sleep-Inducing Peptide)

This peptide is beneficial in reversing some effects of insomnia when used in low doses. As medical doctors become more aware of the dangers of drugs like Ambien, Lunesta, and Trazodone to induce sleep, more peptide use will become mainstream. Long-term use of sleeping pills in general is dangerous because of addictive tendencies as well as their interference with restorative sleep. Sleep is one of the most important processes in slowing down aging. DSIP may also help stimulate testosterone levels.

Anti-Aging Peptides

Peptides not only assist in injury repair and immune modulation, they also have anti-aging benefits. Most doctors are aware that we have for years been looking for peptides that mimic ghrelin or other ways to release growth hormone. HGH has been shown to have great benefits in the field of anti-aging medicine, but the FDA has restricted its use due to their concern about the potential of promoting cellular growth. While there is no real clinical evidence that HGH does have that adverse effect, it is still somewhat restricted for use. Now it is exciting to announce that we have ghrelin-like peptides that work much more efficiently than the original Semorelin with GHRP2 or GHRP 6. CJC 1295 with Ipamorelin stimulates the release of HGH from the pituitary gland as well as increasing HGH secretagogue receptors. One hundred micrograms (100 μg) of CJC 1295 in combination with Ipamorelin taken five to six days a week has a huge impact on improving muscle mass, slowing down body fat, and decreasing oxidation.

IGF-I itself has unique benefits and has been used extensively in HIV positive individuals along with growth hormone to improve muscle mass, appetite, and vitality. Since our focus is on aging/anti-aging medicine, we cannot go into an extensive review of all peptides, so I will leave that for another discussion in future books.

Disease-Fighting Peptides

Even though this book's major concern is on fighting the aging process, I want individuals to be aware of the fact the peptides are now being re-explored for their ability to control certain illnesses. There are so many autoimmune diseases and inflammatory diseases of the bowel and post-traumatic brain disorders that have literally no medicinal pharmacologic treatments. Peptides could be the answer and solution to many of these problems.

Many peptides have emerged as natural compounds that can treat disease of aging. For example:

Cerebrolysin was recently shown to be a more natural means to treat Parkinson's disease and Alzheimer's disease (by reducing amyloid plaques).

CHK-Cu is a potent anti-inflammatory peptide for treating arthritis and inflammatory joint diseases. It also helps repair muscle breakdown after vigorous exercise.

AOD 9044 is effective in fat burning and weight reduction and is a more natural approach to preventing obesity.

IGF-1 (Insulin Growth Factor-1) has benefits in treating HIV–AIDS patients who are experiencing cachexia and muscle-wasting disease.

LL37 confers antimicrobial benefits and represents a natural means to fight infections.

PEG-MGF has been shown to help in muscular dystrophy, AIDS, ALS (amyotrophic lateral sclerosis, also called Lou Gehrig's disease).

Pentosin is used to treat osteoarthritis inflammation.

PT141 boosts libido in both men and women. (Use with caution, however, because it stimulates melanocyte production and therefore should not be used if there is a history of melanoma in the family.)

Selank, when combined with oxytocin and the amino acid theanine, can alleviate depression and wean individuals off the more harmful antidepressants. This is by far one of my favorite additions for those suffering with anxiety and depression. I use this peptide in combination with an adaptogenic herb in the ginseng family, along with an NAD stimulant (nucleotide riboside) nasally to get my patients off the use of drugs that affect their libido and moods.

Semax helps treat children and adults with ADD and ADHD. It also detoxifies the body of heavy metals.

Now that you have insight into the anti-aging benefits of hormones and peptides, let's talk about their practical use—how you can use them in your own Rejuvenation Solution Program.

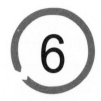

6

Solution:

STRENGTHEN THE HORMONE-PEPTIDE CONNECTION

In 2014, then forty-eight-year-old Rebecca found herself on the verge of plunging headfirst into early aging after undergoing a radical hysterectomy. Her blood pressure was on the rise. She suffered constant anxiety and panic attacks. She had trouble sleeping. Especially unbearable and scary were her heart palpitations. For Rebecca, this time of life was, as she put it, "horrific."

"I was also too extremely exhausted for anything," Rebecca said. "I even stopped doing Pilates, which I loved."

Perhaps even harder to handle than any of these symptoms, though, was Rebecca's sense that she had lost control over her own life. People who are sick often express a feeling of helplessness, but Rebecca wasn't sick. Physiological changes had sent her into a tailspin in which she felt betrayed. "My body," she felt, "had turned against me, and I felt old."

Other doctors had put her on Xanax, an anti-anxiety, anti-depressant drug, and prescription medications for her high-blood pressure. She had been on birth control pills for many years but had recently stopped taking them. Her doctors had scared her into thinking that something serious was wrong with her, and this fear had worsened her anxiety.

Fortunately, tests to pinpoint the cause of the palpitations revealed that she had no coronary artery disease, despite the fact that it ran in her family.

As part of her treatment plan, I suggested that she have her hormone levels tested—and so we did. Those tests revealed that she was clearly in menopause, which had been masked by taking birth control pills for so long.

I knew I could help Rebecca feel better within a few days if she went on a program of bioidentical hormone replacement. I initially prescribed sustained-release progesterone at bedtime. Later, I elected to put her on testosterone cream at night, too. As we were rebalancing her hormones, I also prescribed bioidentical estrogen for a short period of time.

What many practitioners don't understand is that bioidentical hormone treatment can be enhanced with other natural, anti-aging therapies, depending on the patient. In Rebecca's case, I took her off Xanax and replaced it with an adapotogenic herb called Prime One, a derivative of ginseng for a short period of time, and an Ayurvedic herb called Stress Free Emotion twice a day. To help control blood pressure, I put her on a Chinese herb called BP Balance. I taught her to meditate using a mantra that I whispered to her. I instructed her to sit quietly and meditate for five to twenty minutes twice a day.

Another key factor I've learned in treating literally thousands of women in early menopause or even pre-menopause is to consider a process called *methylation*, which I discussed earlier. It is intricately involved in so many key processes: DNA renewal and repair, detoxification, immunity, and nerve protection, among others. If a woman's methylation cycle is off, it can lead to problems with anxiety, depression, and hot flashes.

To check Rebecca's methylation cycle, I ordered a saliva DNA test. I wanted to know what the cause of her anxiety and fatigue was, since her heart evaluation was normal. As I suspected, her test showed me that her methylation was off. This could be corrected through nutrition. I made sure she ate more nutrients high in methyl groups, such as B vitamins and the amino acids methionine and betaine, all found in vegetables and plant proteins. These nutrients help donate methyl groups to proteins, DNA, and other molecules to keep your body detoxifying and functioning well.

I also prescribed 50 billion colonies of a probiotic to take twice a day with meals, as well as instructing her to eat more plant-based nutrition for her prebiotics. I realized I could improve both her sleep and her anxiety with tryptophan and magnesium. Sleep is an amazing remedy for young women who are tired and wired and fearful.

To ease her palpitations and elevated blood pressure, I gave her 100 milligrams of 5-hydroxytryptophan for sleep (5-HTP), 100 milligrams of magnesium sulfate, and a slow-release progesterone, made by a compounding pharmacy. After I restored her progesterone, she no longer needed 5-HTP for sleep.

"Within days, I felt 100 percent better," Rebecca said. "It feels so good to just feel normal—and younger."

For Rebecca, all of the treatments—from taking hormones to correcting her methylation to adjusting her nutrition and more—restored a sense of normalcy.

As Rebecca discovered, you can retain the youthfulness you had in your twenties when you're in your fifties, sixties, and beyond with anti-aging hormone replacement and peptide manipulation. These actions can firm up flabby muscles and skin, reduce your wrinkles, increase your energy, ignite your sex drive, and protect you from diseases of aging. Anti-aging hormones and peptides are an effective way to pick up any part of your system that is flagging with age.

Bioidentical Hormone Replacement

Bioidentical hormones are made from plants, such as the wild yam or soybean plant or other natural substances, and are chemically and functionally identical to human hormones. The wild yam, for example, contains building-block molecules that can be converted in the laboratory into estrogens and other hormones whose molecular structure matches those produced in the body.

Up until menopause and andropause, our bodies make adequate amounts of hormones—and then we age, living in a state of hormone deficiency.

Bioidentical hormones are simply a way to replace sex hormones (estrogen, progesterone, testosterone) for both women and men. The hormones are applied topically to the body, taken orally, or given by injection. The body recognizes them because they are structurally similar to the body's own hormones, and therefore knows what to do with them. Bioidentical hormones bind to hormone receptor sites in the same way that our own hormones do.

Are Bioidentical Hormones Safe?

Yes. They are safe because they bind to hormone receptor sites in the exact same way that your own hormones do, so they do not trigger side effects. Which bioidentical hormones you need, and how much, will depend on your levels—which must be measured through laboratory tests, usually blood tests and/or saliva tests.

With hormones, your treatment may include a cocktail of prescription-only hormones including human growth hormone (HGH), and estrogen and testosterone, often prescribed as gels or creams. I concede that hormone therapy isn't the whole answer, but it can play a vital role in slowing the aging process.

Synthetic Hormones versus Bioidentical Hormones

Prior to the advent of bioidentical hormones, women were prescribed synthetic hormones, manufactured from the urine of pregnant mares, namely the synthetic estrogens Premarin and Provera. Also prescribed was the synthetic progesterone Prempro. These drugs were used in the infamous Women's Health Initiative (WHI). Data from this study was released in 2002. It linked hormone replacement therapy (HRT) to potentially life-threatening consequences:

- 26 percent increase in invasive cancer
- 29 percent increase in myocardial infarctions or death from coronary artery disease
- 41 percent increase in the risk of stroke
- 200 percent increase in the risk of blood clots

The WHI study also confirmed benefits:

- 33 percent decrease in the risk of hip fracture
- 37 percent decrease in the risk of colorectal cancer
- Relief of menopausal symptoms like hot flashes and vaginal atrophy

As a result of these findings, guidelines for HRT use changed, with doctors told to prescribe it only in certain circumstances, and HRT prescriptions plummeted.

But twelve years later, with additional WHI data crunching, women in the WHI who had taken estrogen had a significantly lower rate of invasive breast cancer than did those who had taken placebo. Additionally, they did not have higher risks for heart attacks, blood clots, or strokes. And other follow-up research on women in their fifties suggested that taking estrogen alone might actually protect middle-aged women's hearts.

Other WHI follow-up data revealed that the true trigger for breast cancer and heart problems was synthetic, non-bioidentical progesterone, given as Prempro, progestins, or medroxyprogesterone.

Synthetic hormones are not identical to the human hormone molecule, and do not fit cellular receptors correctly. This is why they account for a multitude of side effects—and why bioidentical hormones are so superior.

I've used bioidentical estradiol and estriol for more thirty-five years, along with a bioidentical form of progesterone, and I have not seen any adverse side effects.

That being said, I always believe that in any woman who has a family history of breast cancer, the postmenopausal use of even bioidentical hormones should be individualized according to the patient's belief system and their acceptance of current knowledge that bioidentical hormones seem safe.

Also, synthetic hormones have a longer half-life in the body, referring to the time it takes for a drug to lose half its strength in the body. The longer the half-life, the more potential there is for side effects. Bioidentical estrogen has a half-life of only twelve hours, whereas synthetic estrogen lingers in the body for approximately forty-five days.

Bottom line: Synthetic products *are not* the same as the hormones your body produces naturally! And women's bodies *do not* naturally produce the same amounts of hormones every day of the month!

Nonetheless, Premarin remains to be the most commonly used estrogen in the United States, even though it is dangerous.

Your Hormone Levels

Most of the anti-aging hormones can be measured with a blood sample usually taken in the early morning. Some of the hormones such as cortisol and DHEA at times are measured more than once a day to see their normal fluctuations. There are also times when, instead of using blood samples, the hormones are measured with tests using saliva samples. Saliva testing is most beneficial to test for hormones that have cyclical production, such as estrogen and progesterone, which cycle each month in preparation for pregnancy. Some hormones like HGH and insulin are measured after a stimulation challenge to see if there is a normal or subnormal production.

Using Bioidentical Hormones

Everyone is different, so whether you need certain bioidenticals or not depends on your hormone levels and health. Nonetheless, here is an overview of bioidenticals, including forms of administration and, in some cases, typical doses.

Thyroid Hormones

These can be supplemented, too, in people who need them. Because there's no bioidentical version of thyroid hormone, I give my patients small amounts of natural desiccated thyroid supplement that comes from a porcine source. It contains all active thyroid hormones, unlike its synthetic pharmaceutical counterpart, and works very well in most people.

If thyroid replacement is required, you definitely want to consider a natural replacement, such as Armour thyroid, Nature Thyroid, or Westhroid, made from desiccated dried pig tissue that contains the T3 and T4 thyroid hormones. These are drug-like substitutes, not herbs, and they are not available over the counter.

Although the dose can vary from 15 to 240 milligrams, I can't recommend a dosage because it depends on testing to determine. A qualified physician can tailor the dosage to the individual.

You can also supplement with the amino acid tyrosine, which can help the thyroid function better. Whenever possible, eat foods rich in iodine, such as sea vegetables, because iodine supports thyroid function.

You do not want to take the synthetic drug, Synthroid. I renamed it SIN-throid because it has serious side effects, including heart palpitations, difficulty breathing, and chest pain.

DHEA

There is some discussion about whether or not oral DHEA is beneficial; however, I find it to be beneficial in enhancing the immune system, as well as improving strength and vitality. The typical dose of DHEA is 25 to 100 milligrams orally in the morning.

For women suffering from chronic fatigue or cortisol imbalances, I might up that dosage to 100 to 300 milligrams of DHEA.

If you are a woman taking DHEA, however, discontinue its use if you experience dry skin, acne, or hair growth.

Cortisol

Bioidentical cortisol exists, but it is a very short-acting hormone, lasting about three to five hours total per dose. Its effects are usually felt very quickly—usually within five to fifteen minutes. If the dose is correct, you'll feel better, calmer, more focused, and more able to cope, with improved energy and stamina to make it through the day.

However, bioidentical cortisol is not usually practical and can have side effects, including further cortisol imbalances. An alternative to bioidentical cortisol is an adrenal extract, available as a supplement.

Testosterone

Testosterone is the most common form of natural hormone replacement in men. Men with declining testosterone levels have a wide range of symptoms, including erectile dysfunction, fatigue, and loss of libido that come on gradually.

Women often require bioidentical testosterone, too. It is often believed that estrogen is the protective hormone for the heart. Testosterone, however, has more receptors in the heart muscle; therefore, the use of testosterone in women seems to be more protective than estrogen to prevent cardiovascular disease.

In women, bioidentical testosterone comes in a cream to be applied to the body, usually on the wrists, or as an injection once or twice a week. If given in too high of a dosage to a woman, testosterone can cause hair growth on the face and even hair loss from the scalp.

ASK DR. BOB: Does taking bioidentical testosterone increase a man's risk of prostate cancer?

The medical profession has offloaded this misconception for years. Dr. Morgentaler at Mass General Hospital in Boston has done extensive research to show that testosterone is safe, has no adverse effects on increasing PSA (Prostate Screening Antigen), and can be used safely in men who have existing prostate cancer. Dr. Morgentaler's research has categorically disproven the myth that taking testosterone causes prostate cancer.

The bioidentical form of testosterone is testosterone cypionate. There are other longer-acting forms of testosterone, such as propionate and enanthate, that can have longer-term uses, and many physicians are now using combinations of cypionate along with these.

A common delivery method for men is with testosterone pellets. This requires a minor incision in the buttocks to implant the pellets. I prefer intramuscular biweekly testosterone injections over pellets because injections appear to be more effective. The typical dose to maintain health, vitality, libido, and sex drive is 80 to 160 milligrams weekly.

Testosterone does not always improve sexual function, however. There are other reasons for sexual dysfunction. These include the presence of type 2 diabetes or cardiovascular disease; the overuse of medications such as blood pressure drugs, antidepressants, beta blockers, and statins (which lower cholesterol—the building block of all hormones). With the increased use of these medications in men in particular, I find it necessary to include nitric oxide supplementation (which dilates blood vessels for better blood flow) to improve quality of erections.

Men at any age with declining testosterone should avoid eating animal proteins, such as dairy foods and meat. They are laden with artificial hormones, which interfere with the production of the body's natural hormones. This leads to low sperm counts and low testosterone.

Finally, there are a growing number of young men who have low testosterone levels below 300, who can be treated either with human chorionic gonadotropin (HCG) or Clomid on a short-term basis.

Estrogen

With age, a woman's body produces less estrogen, and this natural hormone can be replaced with bioidentical hormone replacement therapy. The actual natural hormones that are used are 17 beta-estradiol, estrone, and estriol, applied as a cream to the skin. (Estradiol is the form of estrogen that decreases at menopause.) These are also the most studied as far as the positive effects.

In women who experience continued vaginal dryness, low libido, or dry skin and who do not have an increased risk of family history of breast cancer, I prescribe Biest Cream 80 percent/20 percent–estradiol estriol.

Progesterone

Bioidentical progesterone taken as an oral supplement in a slow-release capsule offers protection to the uterus in women who are still menstruating, as well as to breast tissue. It also protects bones, lubricates the vagina, promotes sound sleep, and fights aging.

Generally, I prescribe a dose of 100 to 300 milligrams of slow-release progesterone. I follow a woman's progress on a weekly basis to see if I need to add in bioidentical estrogen, especially if she is peri-menopausal or post-menopausal.

Insulin

Bioidentical insulin does not exist; however, insulin can be balanced and regulated naturally by diet and exercise, unless you've been diagnosed with type 1 or severe type 2 diabetes and need to take insulin injections.

A condition called insulin resistance, in which the body does not use insulin properly and it builds up in the blood, can be addressed by not eating processed carbohydrates, reducing all carbohydrates in general, and by consuming natural, whole, organic foods. Exercise, particularly strength training, is important, too, because it helps muscle cells respond to insulin better.

HGH

HGH is one bioidentical hormone that must be delivered by injection. The amount of HGH you will need in each dose, and how long you will need to be on HGH therapy will vary from patient to patient. Your course of HGH treatment is based on the results of your initial lab analysis, and like all bioidentical therapy, is tailored to your specific needs for optimum anti-aging results.

Some people have heard that supplementing with HGH can cause cancer. There is currently no evidence pointing toward this. HGH, however, does cause cellular growth. Therefore, in people who currently have cancer, it is suggested that they not use exogenous HGH. If someone has a family history of cancer, I would strongly suggest that using growth-hormone releasing peptides instead of HGH is a better approach to obtain the benefits of HGH without worry of side effects.

If you take HGH, the usual dosage depends on your sex, body fat percentage, and age, among other factors. Generally, a safe dosage is 1 unit daily six days a week. Higher dosages may be required under certain medical conditions.

Melatonin

Melatonin is available over the counter as a nutritional supplement. A typical dosage for treating insomnia is 1 to 5 milligrams of melatonin at bedtime. Because the daily production of melatonin tends to decline after age thirty by about 0.5 milligrams every decade, a dose of 0.5–2.0 milligrams may be relevant as an anti-aging approach.

Melatonin is a very powerful rejuvenating hormone that is made by the brain from a neuroendocrine pathway. If we are ever able to measure melatonin levels clinically, it may become one of the best *age predictors*. It is really not a sleep aid, but works through enzymes that promote sleep. Some people are very sensitive to melatonin and have very bad dreams when they take it because of a missing or sluggish SNP enzyme.

These bioidentical hormone therapies, in my opinion, are well tolerated, provide symptom relief, and can address many of the health needs as well as reverse the aging process. You'll obtain most of these hormones at compounding pharmacies, which customize the formula as prescribed by your physician. Traditional pharmacies only distribute drugs that are manufactured by corporate pharmaceutical companies.

If you are unsure about whether you want to pursue bioidentical hormone replacement, speak to your doctor about your concerns. Together, you can develop an anti-aging plan that fits your needs.

Harness the Power of Peptides

Hormone replacement therapy is one necessary means to slow down the aging process. Peptides now bring us to the next and perhaps the most recent benefits of the anti-aging medicine solutions.

There are now peptides that we can safely use in anti-aging medicine to treat inflammation and oxidation and repair DNA and raise telomerase levels. We are finding more benefits every day, so hold onto your hats as I cover this next section.

By the way, if this book were about peptides it would literally have to be rewritten weekly to revise it. That is how fast this scientific process is moving. Here a brief look at how peptides are currently administered:

Some of the peptides that can help mitigate or reverse this aging process are:

Ghrelin. This peptide is currently not available for clinical use, but you can maintain healthy concentrations of this peptide in your blood. For one thing, if you are overweight, you'll want to get to your ideal weight through proper nutrition and exercise. Ghrelin concentrations in blood are low in obese people, compared to lean subjects. To further normalize ghrelin levels, maintain a nutrition program that is high in plants and fruits. Another way to manipulate ghrelin is to increase the duration or the intensity of your exercise sessions. Recent data suggest that prolonged exercise produces an increase in ghrelin levels. This may be the mechanism that causes HGH to rise after exercise.

Sermorelin, Tesamorelin, CJC 1295, and Examorelin. The dose varies from 100 to 500 micrograms (μg) six days a week to allow the body and the pituitary gland to recover. These peptides can be taken either subcutaneously or intramuscularly.

GHRP 2, GHRP 6, Ipamorelin. The typical dose by injection it is 100–300 μg of these GH secretagogues.

BPC 157. This peptide can be taken orally or injected subcutaneously. The average dose is 500 mcg orally once or twice a day; 300–600 mcg once or twice a day.

Alpha 1 (TA1) and Thymosin Beta 4 (TB4). TA1 is injected subcutaneously 0.15 mL (450 µg) daily, and may be used in combination with TB4, especially to treat autoimmune diseases. TB4 is injected subcutaneously 0.25 mL (750 µg) daily or twice-daily.

DSIP (Deep-Sleep-Inducing Peptide). This is administered subcutaneously or nasally, 100 µg dose, usually once a day.

Cerebrolysin. This is administered in oral doses of 215 mg or can be injected 215 mg intramuscularly for a four-week course. This can be given at 215 mgs orally for 40 days as well as by injection.

CHK-Cu. Can be given in a transdermal cream 5% 2 pumps daily or injected 10 mgs/ml and injected 0.2 cc. subcutaneously 20 mg.

AOD 9044. This can be used as a transdermal cream or an injectable for twenty days.

IGF-1 (Insulin Growth Factor-1). This peptide can be taken orally 500 µg daily.

Selank-peptide. This is given in a dose of 750 µg nasally every day or 300 mcg/kg body weight for post-traumatic stress disorder and ADHD.

Semax. This is a class of peptides usually administered nasally at 750 µg up to 300 mg dose daily for ADHD and post-traumatic stress.

RG3/NR/B12. This nasal spray is used to improve brain function. The dose is one spray in each nostril once or twice a day.

This information is just the beginning of our investigation into the world of peptides as a valuable weapon against both the aging process as well as in preventing disease.

ASK DR. BOB: Will peptides replace bioidentical hormones?

No, but I do believe that in the future as we identify improvements in the overall signaling effect of peptides we may find that it is unnecessary to use bioidentical hormones to achieve cellular protection. The currently available peptides are not going to accomplish the same thing that bioidentical hormones do. Therefore, I often use a combination of bioidentical hormones and peptides to improve energy, decrease inflammation, improve mental clarity, and reduce the oxidative stress of the aging process.

I remain excited about peptides—for two reasons. First, they may alter the course of many diseases. There are 7,000 peptides in the human body—so just imagine the possibilities for treatment and possibly cures. Second, peptides are natural cellular mechanisms that signal the body to repair itself, decrease inflammation, and improve the underlying mitochondrial dysfunction in most diseases.

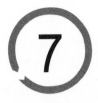

SHORTENED TELOMERES

Humankind has always been searching for the Fountain of Youth in order to prolong life and stay young. We may be getting closer to that answer, and one of those answers lies in unraveling the mystery of telomeres and telomerase. Whole books have been written on both, as if they are the only Fountain of Youth. But I take a different stance: They are just one of the seven causes of aging, and they interact synergistically with the other six—a fact that many experts fail to explain. *Let's pick that idea up* and run with it.

What Are Telomeres?

Telomeres are specialized strands of DNA, located at the end of chromosomes. Their length has been associated with the aging of the cells. Shortened telomeres, for example, accelerate aging and disease.

Once scientists discovered telomeres, it became a scientific quest to learn how to control the fate of each cell of our body—and slow its rate of aging. One of the first discoveries about telomeres was that environmental factors can shorten them and therefore accelerate aging. These factors include poor nutrition, food additives, GMOs, smoking, obesity, diabetes, and exposure to heavy metals and toxins, chronic infections such as hepatitis C, irradiation, air pollution, and contaminated water supplies. Specifically, these factors shorten telomeres, as well as increase DNA mutations, which also shorten telomeres.

Chromosome

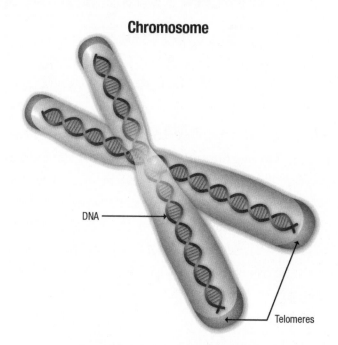

DNA

Telomeres

Telomeres and Aging

Telomeres protect the ends of the chromosomes from deteriorating and shortening, without damaging the genes. So basically, telomeres protect the DNA from being damaged.

Every time a cell replicates (duplicates), however, telomeres shorten. When telomeres become too short, the cell can no longer replicate.

This phenomenon was first described by Leonard Hayflick in 1965. His so-called *Hayflick limit* essentially says that every cell in the body can only repair itself if there are long telomeres to protect the end of the DNA. The lack of protection causes *senescence* (old age), which is the aging of the cell and also aging of the organism. When an organism, say a human being, cannot repair itself by replacing damaged cells or organs, it eventually malfunctions, disease occurs, and death ensues.

The mechanism of repair and protection of the telomere is under the control of an enzyme called *telomerase*. Enzymes work by activating certain chemical reactions in the cells and the body in general; turning food into energy in the cell, for example, requires many different enzymes. Most of these have a specific job description. The job description of *telomerase* is to protect the telomere from shortening, while still performing its function of repairing damaged cells.

When a child is conceived, telomeres carry about 15,000 DNA base pairs. Because telomerase can't keep up with rapid cell division in the womb, they shrink to about 10,000 base pairs at birth.

Once we leave our teens, we lose fifty base pairs a year. In our "golden years," our telomeres drop below about 5,000 base pairs. Cells then may lose their ability to divide, often becoming senescent, unable to do the work they were designed to do but good at doing things like releasing inflammatory chemicals that harm nearby tissue. Or, they may succumb to cell death.

Anti-Aging Pioneers: Elizabeth H. Blackburn, PhD, and William Andrews, PhD

Professor Blackburn discovered the molecular nature of telomeres and co-discovered with a lab assistant the enzyme telomerase in a protozoan, an achievement that won them a Nobel Prize. Since then, our picture of human telomeres and telomerase has sharpened considerably.

Blackburn and her research team at the University of California, San Francisco continued to work with various cells (including human cells) with the goal of further understanding telomerase and telomere biology.

A molecular biologist and gerontologist, William Andrews has worked as a medical researcher since 1981, focusing on cancer, heart disease, and inflammation, though his passion has always been aging. In the early- to mid-1990s, while at the Geron Corporation, Andrews led the research to discover both the RNA and protein components of the human enzyme telomerase.

In 1999, Andrews founded the biotech company Sierra Sciences in Reno, Nevada, to capitalize on his discoveries at Geron, with the specific goal of curing human aging.

Telomerase and the Ageless Body

There is evidence that telomerase can lengthen telomeres and slow down the aging at least at the cellular level. It has been proposed that if we increase the length of our telomeres, we would prolong the human life span and prevent most diseases, even cancer. Prolongation of the life span has not been proven in humans, but telomere lengthening has reversed signs of aging in mice.

Studies in humans have identified a gene(s) on chromosome 4 that may promote longevity and seems to be prevalent in centenarians. Thus, there may be a genetic component to both telomeres and telomerase. This theory has yet to be proven, however, but it does pose interesting anti-aging implications. In the meantime, the search for products and behaviors that keep telomerase levels high seems to have promise for future research.

One of the largest studies to date on telomeres shed some light on telomeres' effect on a person's longevity potential. Researchers collected saliva samples and medical records of more than 100,000 participants. Their findings showed that shorter-than-average telomere length was associated with a boost in mortality risk—even after adjusting for life- style factors like smoking, alcohol consumption, and education that are linked to telomere length.

The study found that individuals with the shortest telomeres, or about 10 percent of the study's participants, were 23 percent more likely to die within three years than those with longer telomeres.

A study in the July 7, 2010, *Journal of the American Medical Associ- ation* highlighted the correlation between cancer and short telomeres: People with shorter-than-average telomeres had three times the risk of developing cancer and eleven times the risk of dying from it.

Because of all this, the lengthening of telomeres with telomerase or embryonic stem cell production should be the target for many types of therapy, including anti-aging and anti-cancer therapies. After all, telo- merase interventions would preserve the immune system and organs— unlike chemotherapy and radiation, both of which have more side effects than cures. They (chemo and radiation) destroy healthy cells, deplete telomerase, and attack the immune system. This potentially means that chemo and radiation would essentially shorten the life span!

Testing Your Telomeres

There is now a test available that can measure your telomeres. You simply order a telomere test kit from a testing organization. Once you receive it, take a saliva swab or a blood sample, send the kit back to the company, and wait to receive your results.

Remember, at birth, you have 10,000 DNA base pairs. Your biologic age is a factor of how many based pairs are remaining. As I explained, as soon as you are born, your telomeres shorten, and you gradually lose pairs over your lifetime.

The telomere test can measure your based pairs, so its primary benefit is in the information it provides to you regarding biological age and
telomere length. This information allows you to make adjustments to
your lifestyle that can lead to better health and a longer life. The cost of
these tests begin at around $89 to measure *average telomeres* and about
$300 to $400 to identify *short telomeres* and predict true biologic age.

I favor measurement of short telomeres since, in my opinion, average
telomere length is often misleading. Life Length, a Spanish company,
offers the only tests with the accuracy that I believe should be used for
measuring telomere length. Once you know your telomere or biologic
age, you can decide how and when to retest.

Some of you may say, "I do not want to know if my telomeres are short!"

Knowing telomere length, however, can also be used to let you know
if you are at risk for heart disease, type 2 diabetes, and even certain cancers because these are associated with short telomeres. If you have this
information, you can take actions to change your lifestyle and ultimately
lengthen your telomeres. Doing so is the essence of epigenetics—changing your actions, behavior, or lifestyle to change whether or not a gene
expresses itself in a harmful way.

Because telomeres can predict how you age, why wouldn't you want
to know your telomere length? Wouldn't you want to take actions to
lengthen your telomeres and by doing so, lengthen your life and change
the quality of your later years so that you are fit and independent?
Think about it.

Being as vigorous as possible as we age should be the goal for everyone. And this is relatively easy to accomplish. A few examples: longer
telomeres are positively associated with the consumption of legumes,
nuts, seaweed, and fruits, and negatively associated with the consumption of alcohol, red meat, excess sugar, and processed meat.

Then there's the effect of exercise on telomere length. Research
shows that high-intensity aerobic exercise, such as cycling, boosts

skeletal muscle telomeres more than moderate exercise. Exercise also stimulates telomerase activity.

Stress will shorten your telomeres, too. In a study of women who reported high psychological stress, their telomeres were shorter.

What's more, when you practice the antioxidant and anti-inflammatory solutions I outlined in chapters 2 and 4, you will lengthen your telomeres. Telomeres are very susceptible to oxidation and inflammation—which is a huge reason for eating foods high in antioxidants, taking antioxidant supplements, and following my anti-inflammatory protocol.

There are so many solutions you can apply to protect and lengthen your telomeres. That's where we are headed next.

Solution:

TELOMERASE ACTIVATORS

Consider the lives of two people. One is Gracie F., a sixty-one-year-old woman who works long hours, rarely exercises, and takes antidepressants for depression and anxiety. She drinks one to two glasses of wine or vodka daily. She does not meditate, although she prays regularly. She has adopted children and grandchildren, and family is very important to her.

In 2011, Gracie was diagnosed with colorectal cancer (cancer of the large lower portion of the bowel) and underwent chemotherapy and radiation. Thankfully, the treatments worked, and she has been cancer-free for nearly six years.

After her bout with cancer, Gracie was motivated to stay healthier and resist the effects of aging as much as she could. To see where she stood, Gracie had her telomeres measured. Tests showed that Gracie had the telomeres of a sixty-four-year-old woman, and the health of one as well. She was older than her chronological age. (The human body has two different ages: a chronological age and a biological age. Chronological age refers to the actual number of years you've been alive, while biological age refers to how old you seem, based on your health and the length of your telomeres.)

The other person is me, so I'm going to use myself as a mini-case. I have been exercising since I was eight years old. I swim, bike, or run almost daily. I lift weights and do yoga on occasion. I've been a vegan for most of the past thirty-two years of my life. I drink no alcohol. I have been meditating with Transcendental Meditation for almost thirty years, twice a day. I've studied spirituality since the age of twenty; I have a profound belief in God and have explored everything from Kabbalah to the Hindu Dhammapada. I have a fairly high-stress job, but I love it and do not consider it "work." I have five grown children and twelve grandchildren and relish my life and family.

When I was seventy-one, I had my telomeres measured, and my biological age was estimated to be sixty-three.

Why do you think that one person appears to be almost a decade younger than his or her stated age and the other is a few years older than that age? The difference between Gracie and me boils down to telomeres—whether they're long or short—but also on lifestyle. Lifestyle definitely affects telomeres; it's all related. If lifestyle and behaviors are unhealthy, the aging process accelerates, and people have a greater risk of developing serious diseases, such as heart disease and cancer.

What prevents telomeres from shortening is an enzyme called telomerase (te-LAW-mer-ace). It even appears to lengthen them if enough of the enzyme is generated. Scientists are optimistic that telomerase represents a way to reestablish organ health and reverse aging.

This has already been observed in a 2010 Harvard University–based study in which old, dying mice, deficient in telomerase, were given the enzyme to lengthen their telomeres. In these animals, telomere shortening provoked shrinking of tissues, depleted stem cells (cells that can self-heal the body), promoted organ failure, and impaired tissue healing, according to this study. But when telomerase was reactivated, the length of the telomeres in old mice reduced these forms of damage and halted the degeneration of multiple organs, including the testes, spleen, intestines, and even brain cells. The old mice recovered their health and became sexually active.

This evidence suggests that damaged or shortened telomeres are associated with the lack of telomerase. Reactivation of telomerase, in turn, literally reversed aging. As a result of findings like this, there is a vigorous effort going on worldwide to develop regenerative strategies designed to restore telomere integrity.

Science will continue to plow this territory. In the meantime, there are many strategies you can take now to activate telomerase, protect your telomeres, and even lengthen them. I use these strategies myself, so let's pick it up from here.

Harness the Power of Plants

A very effective way to activate telomerase is to eat the way I recommend: more vegetables and fruits—essentially, a plant-based diet. It supplies a lot of fiber, which has been linked with longer telomeres. This type of diet also keeps your weight down and cures chronic inflammation, both telomere-friendly strategies. It is low in animal protein, too, foods shown in studies to reduce telomere length.

There's more: A plant-based, low-meat diet is high in antioxidants, such as vitamins C and E. These nutrients not only neutralize free radicals, but they also slow damage to telomeres, and they do this by picking up the activity of telomerase. This was observed in a study of the Mediterranean-style diet—high in olive oil, vegetables, and fish. People who followed this dietary pattern had longer telomeres and higher telomerase activity, so it's no wonder that so many Greeks and Italians are long-lived.

Also, something as simple as drinking tea is an anti-aging measure that could turn back the clock by as much as five years. A Chinese study of 2,006 men and women discovered that drinking at least three cups of either green or oolong tea daily was associated with longer telomeres. In fact, those longer telomeres were equivalent to being biologically five years younger! Green tea is rich in epigallocatechin gállate (EGCG), a potent antioxidant that is linked to telomerase activity.

The foods and dietary pattern I recommend to fight aging are covered in chapters 12 and 13. If you follow my recommendations, you'll go a long way toward activating telomerase and protecting your telomeres.

Supplement to Boost Telomerase

In addition to healthy nutrition and lifestyle, certain supplements appear to protect telomeres and stimulate telomerase activity. Here's a rundown:

Omega 3s

Available from fish and plant sources, these beneficial fats are an integral component of the traditional Mediterranean diet, and they may be one of the reasons why this diet is associated with longer telomeres and longer life.

Omega 3s appear to slow brain aging, too. In an Australian study, researchers recruited thirty-three men and women sixty-five years of age and older. All had been diagnosed with mild cognitive impairment, a prelude to Alzheimer's disease. The volunteers were given one of three different supplements each day for six months: 1,670 milligrams of eicosapentaenoic acid (EPA) and 160 milligrams of docosahexaenoic acid (DHA); 1,550 milligrams of DHA and 400 milligrams of EPA (DHA is the most potent omega-3; from it, your body can make EPA, which has heart-health benefits); or 2,200 milligrams of linoleic acid, an omega-6 fat found in corn and soybean oils.

The researchers observed that there was telomere shortening in all three groups—a finding chalked up to the older age of the participants. Even so, people who had the highest levels of the omega-3 fat DHA in their blood had the least telomere shortening. In contrast, telomeres shortened the most in people who took the omega-6 linoleic acid.

Dosage: Taking omega-3 fatty acid supplements is a good strategy to reduce telomere shortening. My recommendation is to supplement daily with 3,000 milligrams of plant-based ALA (alpha linoleic acid) from clary sage oil. This form of omega 3 is your body's best friend, since EPA and DHA made from clary sage can cross the blood-brain barrier and improve both cognition and repair of neurons in the brain. Other sources of omega-3s do not have this function.

Folic Acid

This is a B vitamin found naturally in green leafy vegetables and legumes. It protects the body against the effects of homocysteine, an amino acid that is toxic to telomeres, impairing their ability to mend damaged DNA (this process is known as methylation). Fortunately, folic acid suppresses the accumulation of homocysteine and thus guards telomeres from its harmful effects.

Dosage: Plant-based nutrition delivers adequate folic acid (known as folate in food form), as does supplementing daily with a multivitamin tablet. Multivitamins usually contain 400–1,200 micrograms of folic acid. Supplement with a daily multivitamin/mineral tablet (preferably an antioxidant formulation), adhere to a plant-based diet, and you'll supply your body with ample folic acid. Because it is a critical component of the methylation process, I recommend measuring the blood levels of folic acid on a regular basis to be sure they are adequate.

Carnosine

Found exclusively in animal tissues, carnosine is an amino acid that appears to have the ability to reverse the aging process of cells. It is a powerful antioxidant, working against free radicals that are responsible for aging. In our youth, carnosine shields us from the onslaught of oxidation, glycation, DNA damage, and other reactions that injure tissues and cripple organs. The latest word on carnosine is that it is considered a telomerase activator because it protects telomeres. Scientists first observed this several years ago when they treated human cells in lab dishes with carnosine. It reduced telomere damage and slowed down the rate of telomere shortening.

Dosage: As we grow older, carnosine levels in the body decline, leaving us vulnerable to the signs of aging and the diseases of aging. You can't get carnosine from plant foods—another reason to supplement. The daily dose of carnosine starts at 500 milligrams.

Vitamin D

This vitamin is a prohormone, meaning that it amplifies, or changes an existing hormone in the body, and it appears to protect telomeres. Researchers at Georgia Regents University, Augusta, asked thirty-seven overweight volunteers to supplement with 2,000 IU of vitamin D or a placebo (look-alike pill) daily for sixteen weeks. The supplement takers had nearly a 20 percent spike in the activity of telomerase.

There is now very strong evidence that total vitamin D in the blood should have a range of 50–80 ng/ml. Genetically speaking, some people do not metabolize vitamin D adequately, generally because cellular receptors for this nutrient are not working up to par—a malfunction that can be tested. If you're among this group, you may require more vitamin D than other people.

Dosage: Supplement with vitamin D3 (the most active form of this vitamin), and take 2,000–10,000 IUs daily or 50,000 IUs weekly.

Magnesium

Magnesium is required for more than three hundred biochemical reactions in the body. It helps preserve healthy muscle and nerve function, keeps your heart rhythm steady, bolsters immunity, and upholds bone strength. Magnesium also helps keep blood sugar levels in check, supports normal blood pressure, and is involved in energy metabolism. No wonder there is an increased interest in the role of magnesium in preventing and managing disorders such as hypertension, cardiovascular disease, and diabetes. Now magnesium is being trumpeted by many as a major anti-aging supplement. Studies using human cells have found that a low bodily supply of magnesium shortens telomeres and accelerates aging. Consider: Two-thirds of Americans are deficient in magnesium, and I believe this may promote the aging of millions of people.

Dosage: I suggest taking 200 to 400 milligrams of magnesium daily, preferably at night, because this mineral helps with sleep.

Consider This Rejuvenating Telomerase Activator

There is a nutritional supplement you can purchase without a prescription called TA-65. It is a naturally occurring molecule derived from the astragalus plant, a powerful antioxidant that shows anti-aging promise in research. In a study with mice, it was shown to activate the telomerase enzyme, lengthen critically short telomeres, rescue cells in various organ systems, and improve health span (the number of healthy years you experience). The supplement even improves skin texture.

As for human studies, research indicates that people who take TA-65 have a decrease in blood pressure, cholesterol, and fasting glucose, as well as an increase in bone density. It also restores an aging immune system.

Dosage: The recommended dosage is 2–6 capsules daily, based on the results of your telomere testing. It can cost anywhere from $100 to $400. The testing company I recommend is Life Length in Madrid, Spain.

If your test reveals the highest number of short telomeres, for example, you'd supplement at the higher range. It works best when you employ the other telomerase-activating strategies covered here.

Add Four-Plus Years to Your Life: Kick Your Soda Habit

Americans drink a lot of soda, a habit that's hazardous to your health, waistline, and age. In fact, a Yale survey reported that a majority of Americans understand that soda is bad for them. That's good, because it is. But despite this, a Gallup poll revealed that 48 percent of surveyed Americans—nearly half!—drink soda on a daily basis.

Well, now comes the news that soda drinking might shorten your telomeres, according to University of California, San Francisco, researchers who found in a new study that drinking sugary drinks was associated with cellular aging.

Their study discovered that telomeres were shorter in the white blood cells of 5,309 survey participants, aged forty to sixty-five, who reported drinking soda daily. The researchers calculated that daily consumption of a twenty-ounce soda was associated with 4.6 years of additional biological aging! The findings were reported online October 16, 2014, in the *American Journal of Public Health*. This is the first demonstration that soda is associated with telomere shortness. Further, although they studied only adults here; it is possible that soda consumption might be associated with telomere shortening in kids, too.

What about diet sodas? They're just as bad. Although there have been no studies to my knowledge on diet sodas and telomere length, these beverages can damage health. A review study of artificial sweeteners, which are an ingredient in diet sodas, noted that these sweeteners may be connected to the risk of cancer, diabetes, heart disease, and kidney disease, headaches, depression, neurological problems, behavioral and cognitive effects, and the risk of preterm delivery.

There's really nothing redeemable about drinking soda of any type. It is linked to all sorts of health problems that will make you age faster: osteoporosis, obesity, stroke, high blood pressure, diabetes, prostate cancer, and a list of other issues as long as both of my arms.

For many people, soda drinking is a fierce habit to break. My suggestions:

Make up your mind. Getting off soft drinks starts in your head. You've got to make a firm commitment in your mind to give them up. This means a strong "want to" in order to make it happen.

Stock up on alternatives. Don't purchase any more soft drinks (not even diet drinks); don't even have them around. Have alternatives available instead: iced green tea or water enhanced with lemon, oranges, strawberries, or cucumbers.

Make water your go-to refresher. Have non-plastic water bottles handy in your refrigerator and at your desk, and every time you leave the house, take a bottle with you. If water is readily available, you'll be more likely to get into the water-drinking habit.

Drink a glass of water first. If your thirst drives you toward the vending machine to grab a soft drink, fill up a glass of ice water or swill a bottle of cold spring water first.

People drink sodas out of habit or because they're thirsty. You can drink some water first to help interrupt this behavior. Then see if you still want a soda. I bet you won't. A lot of times, people drink soda just because they're bored or thirsty, and that's what's available or what they're used to.

Avoid soda triggers. Drinking soft drinks is like many habits: You tend to drink them in certain places or situations, such as restaurants with certain foods, in the morning upon waking up, or as part of an afternoon snack. Analyze your soda-drinking patterns and identify what triggers them. Substitute healthier beverage options in these situations.

Cold turkey or not? Although I'd like to see you go cold turkey on sodas, you may have to wean yourself off them—especially if you gulp down multiple servings a day. Try cutting back to one a day for a week. Then ease off to two or three a week, until you're down to drinking zero soft drinks, and you're off them for good. In many soda drinkers, adjusting gradually helps lead to permanent habit change.

Move More

Regular exercise is another way to lengthen your telomeres, and we know this for a fact because athletes tend to have longer telomere lengths than non-athletes. Further, a British study found those who exercised more had longer telomeres. Why does exercise produce this positive effect? Scientists theorize that it reduces harmful chronic inflammation, and in doing so, improves telomere length.

What kind of exercise is best for telomere preservation and lengthening? Answer: anything that gets you moving! And you don't have to be an athlete; moderate exercise is good for your telomeres. As for the exact form of exercise, studies have been done with both aerobic exercise and strength training, all showing that physical activity of any type is key.

Even just getting up from your favorite chair or your desk will protect your telomeres and possibly extend your life span, one study suggests. Research in the *British Journal of Sports Medicine* reported that reducing sedentary activity appeared to lengthen telomeres. The researchers, from the Karolinska Institute in Stockholm, analyzed telomeres in the blood cells of predominantly sedentary and overweight people in their late sixties. They found that the more the people reduced their sitting time, the longer their telomeres. So, if you stand more and exercise more, you'll be healthier and more youthful than if you live a life of physical inactivity.

Stress Less

Pioneering research has found that being under serious, chronic stress can have a direct effect on telomere length by reducing the effectiveness of telomerase. I've seen powerful evidence that regular sessions of tension-melting meditation can make a big difference. One study, published in the August 2013 issue of the journal *Brain, Behavior, and Immunity* supports my own observations. It found that women who were experienced in meditation practices had significantly longer relative telomere length than women who did not meditate. There is an ever-growing body of research that has drawn the same conclusion, so I'm convinced that meditation can be very effective as an anti-aging measure.

I address the relationship between stress and anti-aging in chapters 13 and 14. But let me emphasize here: Managing stress begins with understanding why you're stressed, then taking action to do something about it. You might choose to switch to a less demanding job, shorten your work hours, seek professional help for personal conflicts or financial problems, or change your lifestyle so that you live the way you want to, or in a way you find worthwhile.

There is so much you can do to manage stress and keep it from cutting your life short: exercise, relaxation therapy, and focused meditation, among other techniques. Whatever course of action you take, you can eliminate or at least minimize telomere-shortening, age-stealing stress by examining the conflict, finding its root, and ending it by changing the way you look at it. Any form of stress management that you use will make you happier, healthier—and younger.

Be Happy

When I was thirty-five, I remember studying physically active centenarians as my role models. There was a lot I learned from them, but one aspect that stood out was that they were optimistic and happy. And no wonder: The cells of people who have suffered depression may age more quickly, a study published in *Molecular Psychiatry* suggests. Dutch researchers compared telomeres in more than 2,400 people with and without depression. They found that the telomeres of people who had been depressed were significantly shorter than those of people who had never battled depression. The results remained even after researchers accounted for a host of lifestyle factors that can also damage DNA and shorten telomeres, such as alcohol abuse and cigarette smoking. They calculated that the telomere shortening in people with a history of depression represented about four to six years of advanced aging!

Psychological Conditions that Shorten Telomeres and Accelerate Aging

---

The effects of chronic, psychological conditions may hasten aging—and pretty quickly. Research has suggested that mental and emotional suffering may cut ten years off your life due to greater risk for inflammation, oxidative stress, physical disease, and death of the body's cells, all of which ultimately shorten life span. Fortunately, psychological treatment, meditation, and certain basic lifestyle changes can help reduce the likelihood of physical harm linked to mental distress. The following conditions have been specifically linked to shortened telomeres:

- Abuse (physical and emotional)
- Anxiety
- Bipolar disorder

- Depression
- Persistent attitude of hostility
- Post-traumatic stress disorder (PTSD)
- Social isolation and loneliness

I'm really not surprised by these findings. Depression wreaks physical havoc on the body. It alters hormones, suppresses immunity, and changes how nerves work. People with a history of depression have greater risks for diseases of aging, including heart disease, type 2 diabetes, dementia, and cancer.

In my practice, I have found that those people who are content and happy with the way they have lived their lives—not necessarily with their accomplishments—are often the longest lived.

If you feel plagued by depression or unhappiness, you'll want to pay special attention to my chapters on stress.

The Cancer-Telomerase Myth

Much of the evidence for activating telomerase is not without controversy. Some doctors are concerned because telomerase activity, by making cells immortal, has been associated with a higher risk of cancer. This is a theory, however, that Elizabeth Blackburn, PhD, who led the pioneering research into telomeres, seems to have adopted.

I became very interested in this issue and wanted to know the truth. I have seen over the years how the medical establishment draws wrong conclusions, which is detrimental to the public. As I delved into it, I discovered the work of Maria Blasco, PhD, the head of cancer research for the Spanish government. She had a completely different take on the cancer-telomerase connection. I wanted to get in touch Dr. Blasco.

At the time of my inquiry, one of my colleagues introduced me to Steven Maitlin, the CEO of Life Length, a company in Spain that was measuring short telomeres with a new technology. I reached out to Mr. Maitlin. He connected me to Dr. Blasco, and my answer to the cancer connection was clarified.

Over the years, I have studied enough mavericks in their respected fields to know that they often have correct answers to scientific dilemmas. Dr. Blasco is one of those mavericks. After studying telomerase in cancer patients, she found that when telomerase was increased in the blood, there was no increased risk of cancer. In fact, telomerase is so powerful in keeping DNA healthy that scientists in America are now using it in tests to fight cancer.

I suspect that you'd love to make it to age eighty, ninety, or one hundred or more with your health and vitality intact, and the optimism to keep living productively. The insights I've shared here will stimulate telomerase and lengthen the telomeres in your cells. Practiced consistently, these strategies can lead to a systemic reversal of your age-related issues. In short, you'll be functioning like a much younger person. With your telomeres lengthened, expect to live longer in better health, with the wisdom to avoid any habits that might interfere with a healthy life span.

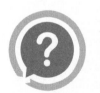

ASK DR. BOB: Can telomere lengthening and telomerase make my skin look younger?

Yes—and there is a revolution going on in the cosmetics industry involving telomerase activators and skin aging. The earliest experiments in this area were done on lab mice. When telomerase was activated in these animals, a couple of things happened. First, there was less skin inflammation. Red or inflamed skin from windburn or sunburn kicks the aging process into high gear, and one result is wrinkles.

Second, the researchers observed that activating telomerase caused cells in the epidermis—the layer beneath the skin surface—to proliferate and thus thicken. When this happens, there is much less wrinkling. Skin normally gets thinner with age, and this was much less obvious. Telomerase activation also plumped up the fat layers just under the skin, too, and of course, this would make skin appear much smoother and more youthful. Finally, older skin is much more prone to injury and heals more slowly. In the mice, this sign of aging was much less pronounced, too.

The TAM-818 Miracle

In 2010, anti-aging researchers at Sierra Sciences, a company founded by Dr. William Andrews, an expert in telomere measurement and testing, screened a molecule now called TAM-818. This stands for Telomerase Activating Molecule; the "818" is a nickname because the original molecule was called 314,818th. It is the strongest telomerase activator yet to be discovered.

TAM-818 has been formulated into a topical skin cream and extensively tested. Results show that it helps to slow signs of aging while significantly reducing the appearance of wrinkles and lines. For example, after thirty days of twice daily use on 100 volunteers, the serum with TAM-818 demonstrated the following:

- The smoothing of forehead wrinkles by 14.04 percent, and likewise crow's feet wrinkles smoothed by 11.07 percent.
- Skin looked firmer by 20.33 percent and skin's elasticity visibly improved by 8.33 percent.

This product is commercially available at *www.tam818.com/buy-online*.

DNA Repair Enzymes

There's more: Cosmetic companies have developed other skin care products formulated with "DNA repair enzymes" from various natural sources. These work by preventing telomere shortening, reversing skin damage from sun exposure, and even preventing the development of skin cancer. They also help thicken skin by inhibiting the development of collagenase, the protein that degrades skin-firming collagen.

Your skin has its own arsenal of naturally occurring enzymes to fix damaged DNA. But with age, the levels of these enzymes drop. It's as though the arsenal has lost its ammunition to fight skin aging, and the wear and tear begins to add up. In a 2013 study published in the *Journal of Drugs in Dermatology*, human skin biopsies taken twenty-four hours after UV exposure showed that DNA repair enzymes, applied topically, fully prevented the degradation of telomeres.

These new skin rejuvenators appear to work even better than topical antioxidants and retinoids (such as Retin-A), which are helpful to skin but do not have the capacity to repair DNA. Topical DNA repair enzymes seem to be the new kid on the anti-aging skin block. If you want healthier, younger-looking, more resilient skin, these products are worth a try.

Cause 5:

PHYSICAL INACTIVITY

If you visit my office desiring to be more youthful and vibrant, I will say the best thing for you is to get on a really good exercise program. Old school as it might seem, exercise is really the best rejuvenation "pill" you can take. With new and solid research, plus what I see in my practice every day, I'm convinced that physical fitness is the ultimate key to extending and improving life. This is no longer a theory of mine; it is scientific fact, backed up by reams of clinical studies.

By how much can exercise extend our lives? To a hundred and twenty years, quite possibly. That's our birthright. But it can be a good 120 years—if you keep moving. It's not lying around in some desolate nursing home.

Sick, Sedentary, and Old!

Unfortunately, many of the problems we experience as we age are not caused by disease but by disuse. In the early twentieth century, the major causes of death were infections, accidents, and complications from war wounds. Fast forward to today: comprehensive reports indicate daily energy expenditure in physical activity has fallen by more than 100 calories a day during the past fifty years.

Maybe you remember as a kid being active, perhaps at school, or when you got home from school and played outdoors with your friends until dinner—or played games or sports all weekend. That's all changed today. Parents now have to set up "play dates"—appointments for their kids to be active and have fun. To me, it's ridiculous and a big reason why we're becoming a nation of couch potatoes.

As society has become less mobile, deconditioning has become a major cause of illness and death. In fact, obituaries should say, "He died from being a couch potato," rather than from heart disease. Is a sedentary lifestyle really such a killer?

Definitely, and the data exist. There's a 2015 study from the *International Journal of Behavioral Nutrition and Physical Activity*, for example, that says watching TV for more than five hours a day kills you.

Heart attacks, strokes, diabetes type 2, obesity, osteoporosis, breast cancer, hypertension, sarcopenia (loss of muscle), and hip fractures are all more prevalent in people who do no regular exercise. Studies have now shown that there are early deposits of a protein called amyloid in the brain of Alzheimer's patients long before they develop symptoms, and that regular exercise is the only therapy that can delay the inevitable cognitive decline associated with the disease.

On a positive note: research shows that regular exercise may reduce the incidence of breast cancer from 1 in 8 to 1 in 20 women. So if you don't exercise, your risk for breast cancer could be higher.

Physical inactivity makes you old before your time. It affects just about every aspect of aging. Too little exercise:

- **Shortens telomeres**—the tips of chromosomes that determine longevity.

- *Is a direct cause of obesity and profoundly affects metabolism.* Less activity requires fewer calories, and we store more food as fat. What's more, there is strong evidence that increased body fat creates more free radicals, primarily ROS and more oxidative stress—the rusting of the body. As I explained in Chapter 1, oxidative stress increases AGEs (accelerated glycation end products), that sticky gooey substance that causes cellular and mitochondrial damage.

  Obesity also shortens telomeres by decreasing telomerase. Unfortunately, physical activity requirements are being eliminated from our schools—which will only fuel the obesity epidemic even more in this country and age us faster than ever.

  This trend, and the rising numbers of sedentary adults, troubles me. It leads to an increased incidence of heart disease and strokes, for one thing. Further, we are now finding that young adults between eighteen and twenty-five are developing heart disease.

- *Increases inflammation, a major cause of the diseases of aging.* People who do not exercise promote the production of inflammatory cytokines—a process that can lead to more oxidative stress to tissues and directly cause cellular damage to the DNA and accelerated aging.

- *Affects anti-aging hormones negatively.* Two of the most affected are HGH and testosterone in both men and women. There is a direct relationship between the release of HGH and an increase in the release of testosterone when you exercise. Both hormones are very important in maintaining muscle, lowering body fat, and even sharpening your brainpower. So when you're inactive, you're missing out on these benefits.

  I'll give you an example. A friend of mine called me about his eighteen-year-old grandson, who weighs 280 pounds, does not exercise, and has no energy. He doesn't sleep well, plays video games, and never goes outside. I was asked to see if I could help.

I was able to obtain the grandson's blood work. His testosterone level was 267 (normal for that age is between 1,000 and 2,000 mg/dl), while his IGF-I level was normal (in the high 200s). His cortisol level was high too—at 20.

After investigating the rest of his blood work, I discovered that his insulin level in a fasting state was 47. It should be less than 5. His was nine times the normal limit! You don't have to be a rocket scientist to see that this young guy was going to develop diabetes.

This chaotic imbalance of hormones explained all his symptoms. This frightening imbalance was caused by one thing: lack of exercise. He didn't need to be given bioidentical testosterone because he was simply too young; it's for men and women over the age of sixty. All he needed to do was get out and move!

His is not an isolated case. Millions of young men and women are suffering the same problems and headed for the same diseases such as diabetes because they are physically inactive.

The Ultimate Rejuvenative Medicine

Physical activity, especially aerobic exercise, increases the amount of oxygen that we consume and deliver to our cells. We can measure health by an exercise test for VO_2 max that I use often to determine how much oxygen you deliver to a kilogram of muscle. This model tells you how healthy your body really is. As I explained in the previous chapter, the higher your VO_2 max, the more oxygenated your tissues are, which slows down the wear and tear from oxidation and inflammation.

Exercise also helps to raise the heart rate and increase blood from the heart. It keeps your muscles strong and lowers body fat. Both benefits affect inflammation, obesity, blood pressure, and oxidation. It also helps to stimulate hormones. Flexible and strong ligaments and tendons prevent falls and osteoporosis and increase bone density.

Individuals who exercise five days a week have lower body fat and lower insulin levels and are less susceptible to infection because of the high antioxidant protection.

If you compared the cells of physically active people with inactive people under the microscope, you'd see that the cells of exercisers look young—with longer telomeres! This is exactly what a breakthrough study of more than 2,400 British twins found: that exercise appears to slow the shriveling of telomeres, perhaps keeping aging at bay.

Studies of women have shown that the only preventive approach to reduce the incidence of breast cancer is to exercise three to five days a week and the incidence is reduced from 1:6 to 1:20. Even a change in diet had less of an effect on breast cancer reduction than exercise.

Mortality from heart attacks is reduced by 50 percent if you exercise for three days a week for three months, and that protection lasts only if you continue to exercise.

Aerobic exercise such as walking, jogging, or swimming stimulates neurons associated with longevity by turning on and increasing a gene called *brain-derived neurotrophic factor*, or BDNF. Researchers have even found that it can reverse memory decline in seniors. They include developing treatments for neurological disorders, as well as growing new neurons to keep the brain pliable and young. The latter is possible by controlling a gene that is key in creating these neurons.

And, strength training revs up the activity of an anti-aging gene known as FOXO. After the age of fifty, strength training to maintain muscle mass will prevent muscle loss and stimulate the FOXO gene. Medically known as sarcopenia, muscle loss is not a disease, but it is one of the major health risks because it leads to weakness and loss of balance control in individuals over the age of sixty.

My Wake-up Call about Exercise

Through most of my childhood and adult life, I was very physically fit. From eight years old until I entered medical school, I played baseball, football, or basketball almost every day of my life. After entering medical school, I was less active. When I entered a seven-year cardiovascular surgical training program, I was almost entirely inactive, although I thought I was healthy.

A friend of mine, Larry Sedenstein, who had a strong family history of heart disease, exercised almost every day. One day he said to me, "I'm afraid that you're just treating heart problems, but not preventing them."

"What do you mean?" I replied. "I'm saving lives everyday by repairing the valves or replacing the coronary arteries to the heart."

"Because my dad died young from heart disease, I realized that my own life could be shortened, too, if I didn't do anything about it. So now I run five to seven days a week, and I think running has lowered my risk of cardiovascular disease," said Larry.

I laughed, "Are you kidding me?"

"I know you have no risk factors, but you are overweight and physically inactive, and you eat junk food all day long. You have a high-stress job. Nor do you realize how lucky you are to have no heart disease running in your family. You still think you're an athlete, but you're a slug!"

Larry suggested that he and I start running together, but I didn't like the idea. Running used to be punishment for me when I was late for college football practice. I hated running!

Later that same week, he invited me to a nine-mile race in which he was competing. There was also a three-mile walk he suggested that I sign up for.

I laughed! Being very competitive, I accepted his invitation—not for the three-mile walk but for the nine-mile run.

Around the same time, I was operating on a thirty-three-year-old man. He was overweight, ate a lot of junk food, and did no exercise. He had a high-stress job, no family history of heart disease, and normal cholesterol. It was like I was operating on myself.

The day of the race, I laced up my Puma shoes and headed to the course track. I was confident. After all, I had been physically fit since the age of eight. Three miles would be a breeze. As you will learn, that was my ego talking, not my body.

Well, at approximately 100 feet in, I noticed that I was out of breath. The next 100 feet were just as painful and as difficult. I was panting so much that I had to jog a little but mostly walk for the remaining 2.8 miles.

That experience was my wake-up call that I was horribly out of shape, physically unfit, and I had to do something about it. So, I practiced running for the next two weeks. It seemed to get easier daily, but I was still unable to run the entire three miles.

I then entered my first 5-K race. After making it across the finish line, four of my medical students remarked that I looked awful, like I was going to have a heart attack.

I felt awful. I couldn't even drive back to my farm. I was too fatigued. I asked my wife to drive us home.

Discouraged, I felt like I would never be physically fit again. Here I was at the age of thirty-four, recognizing that while I had no underlying diseases, I still wasn't healthy.

The words of my dad: "Let's pick it up" echoed in my ears. I started running every day, rain, sunshine, clouds, or snow—slowly at first, then jogging, and on to full-fledged running. Before long I was running a couple of miles and later increased my running to five miles a day. And I went on to compete in marathons. Since then, I have maintained a high fitness level and continue to recognize the value of continuous exercise in reducing the risk of all diseases of aging.

My career then shifted from cardiovascular surgery to prevention of cardiac disease, which was grounded in physical fitness. I also counseled my patients on nutrition, but my major focus was teaching them the value of physical fitness.

Anti-Aging Pioneers: George Sheehan, MD, and Kenneth Cooper, MD

George Sheehan, MD, a cardiologist from Red Bank, New Jersey, changed the course of medicine when he taught the value of exercise to literally thousands of thousands of runners in the mid-'70s to early '90s. He was the editor of *Runner's World* magazine, too.

Sheehan set the world record for the mile at the age of fifty after a sedentary lifestyle as a cardiologist. His belief was that exercise would be the medicine of the future and allow cardiovascular surgeons like me to put away our scalpels.

Kenneth Cooper, MD, the founder of the Aerobics Institute in Dallas, Texas, was the first to coin the term *aerobics*. He also proved that measuring oxygen consumption VO_2 max (see below) could predict the level of fitness as a measurement of health, and the higher your VO_2 max, the less likely you are to develop heart disease.

I was honored to study at his institute in Dallas before I quit cardio-vascular surgery. Cooper and I became friends—a friendship I have cherished over the years. While most people have probably forgotten the founder of the term *aerobics*, Cooper is a giant in the fitness movement and has done more in the field of preventative cardiac disease than any other fitness guru in the United States.

VO_2 Max and Aging

As we get older, our maximal rate of oxygen utilization, or VO_2 max, tends to decline. VO_2 max is a measure of the body's ability to take in oxygen and disperse it to muscles and organs. Oxygen is really your body's fuel. Essentially, it is to your body what gasoline is to a car. Stated as simply as possible, your lungs draw oxygen in, and your heart delivers that oxygen supply to every cell in your body, where it is used to create energy. The more efficient your heart is at delivering oxygen to your body's cells, the more oxygen the body has at its disposal and the more energy you will have. Not only do your heart and lungs get stronger, you will also have less chance of developing any illness because exercise boosts your immune system.

Your VO_2 max depends on many factors, including your exercise program (or lack of one), how many red blood cells you have, how much blood your heart can spew out, your gender, and your age.

Most people reach their peak around their twenties and some in their thirties. But after that, VO_2 max starts to fall by roughly 10 percent each decade. However, if you are over sixty and continue to exercise aerobically, your VO_2 max may decline only by 5 percent per decade, if at all. And, recent data indicates that people in this age range can increase their VO_2 max with exercise to a measurement similar to that of younger persons.

Basically, this means that you can reverse the aging process by increasing and improving your VO_2 max. It is simple to do so; to improve your VO_2 max, perform plenty of aerobic exercises and avoid a couch potato lifestyle.

Research has found that people with a higher VO_2 max live longer, probably because a high VO_2 max has been correlated with a lower risk of cardiovascular disease, according to the American Heart Association (AHA).

And, people who score low on cardiovascular fitness are also more prone to developing certain cancers, such as breast, lung, and gastrointestinal cancers, according to research.

In 1981, I began to measure VO_2 max on all my patients, using a medical device known as a metabolic cart. This testing device is simple and is performed in my office, not at a hospital as many tests require.

Measuring the amount of oxygen that a person consumes during exercise is called VO_2 uptake. The metabolic cart tells the physician or technician an individual's lung capacity, oxygen pulse (VO_2 / Heart Rate = cardiac output), that is, the amount of blood the heart is pumping every minute, leg strength in watts; all while looking at the exercise EKG (electrocardiogram). Over the course of the last thirty-eight years, I have either personally taught or trained physicians to perform this test in thousands of patients to predict their fitness level as well as their health score.

Statistically, if a woman has a VO_2 of under 1.5 L/m during an exercise evaluation, and a man has a VO_2 below 2.0 L/m during exercise, these are clear indicators of the presence of cardiovascular disease and heart dysfunction.

This kind of testing is probably one of the best low-cost procedures to predict levels of health. Anyone who is reading this book should request that his or her physician perform a VO_2 test to tell not only how fit they are, but what the risk of cardiovascular and lung disease is. I feel that this simple procedure can save thousands and thousands of lives and millions of dollars of unnecessary testing.

My advice here: know what your VO_2, your maximum lung capacity, your oxygen pulse, and your body fat percentage. Maintain a VO_2 in excess of 2 L if you are a man; and 1.5 L, if you are a woman. Keep your body fat percentage under 20 percent as a man, and under 22 percent as a woman.

There is no question that physical activity is one of the keys to maximum health and longevity. It just has so many benefits that relate to anti-aging and health: lower blood pressure, a healthier cardiovascular system, weight management, stress relief, reduced inflammation and oxidative stress, better mood, and overall higher energy levels. So, if someone were to ask me, "What is the best way to reduce my risk of premature death?" I'd say becoming as physically fit as you can for the rest of your life.

10

Solution:

ANTI-AGING EXERCISE

When Joe C., a fifty-three-year-old dentist, first came to see me in 1999, he asked if he should have surgery for severe pain in his hip and legs—a condition technically known as *claudication*. It indicates poor circulation in the lower body due to narrowing of the arteries there. The pain prevented him from walking more than a block without having to stop and sit down before resuming his walk. Claudication affects 15 percent of adult Americans over the age of fifty-five and is considered a consequence of aging.

Joe was scheduled for a surgical procedure called a femoral-to-femoral bypass, essentially a graft from a normal artery on the left side to a blocked artery on the right side. As I looked at his arteriogram, a contrast x-ray that shows the blood flow from the aorta to the legs, it revealed a blocked internal iliac artery (the main artery of the pelvis) on his right side and a diseased iliac artery on his left. In other words, the blood flow to both legs was not normal. His surgeon told him if he did not have surgery, he could lose a leg.

As a former vascular and heart surgeon, I was very familiar with the procedure. I read his arteriogram and rendered a stern opinion. I told Joe: "If surgeons do this operation, and it blocks up at any time, you're going to potentially lose both your legs. Do not go through with this operation. It is risky at your age."

I was adamant. I begged him to let me teach him an exercise program I had been using with patients since 1978—a program that had saved 200 people who were scheduled for surgery but ended up not needing it.

"Give me three months. If this program doesn't work for you, I'll advise that you have the surgery, but a totally different type of operation." I said.

The program I designed in 1978 and still use today is called the Claudication Exercise Program. It's based on a combination of cardio activities that generally focus on the lower extremities, frequency (the number of days a week you exercise), your intensity (level of effort), and duration (how many minutes you work out). When I developed this program, very few studies had been done on whether physical activity was effective in increasing pain-free exercise time. Today, there have been hundreds of studies showing that exercise is a simple and effective method of treating patients with claudication.

Joe followed my program exactly as I instructed. After one month, he started to improve, and at the end of three months, he decided to avoid surgery for as long as he could. He continued to exercise using my program.

In 2016, Joe called me, seeking my help again. He shared with me that he was still doing my program. He had a repeat angiogram (a study of blood vessels) in 2004, and his vessels were largely clear of blockages. In fact, he had developed a large number of collaterals to his legs. These are smaller branches of blood vessels that serve as natural bypasses around arteries that are blocked or significantly narrowed. (Essentially, he had done his own nonsurgical bypass).

His reason for the appointment with me was to lose weight because he felt fatigued and suffered insomnia and low libido. He also had shortness of breath while walking on the treadmill and going up and down stairs.

After a thorough physical exam and a VO2 max test, I agreed to work with him on his weight. I informed him that more intense exercise was going to be necessary, and he admitted, "I feel so bad now that I will do anything to get better."

Joe's starting weight was 217 pounds at a body fat of 37 percent, and his blood pressure was too high. I changed his exercise routine to treadmill walking six days a week, a rowing machine three days a week, and the elliptical trainer three days a week. At first, Joe could do only one minute on the rowing machine; now he's up to fifteen minutes. Both his duration and speed on the treadmill have increased significantly, as has his performance on the elliptical. He also changed his nutrition. I started him on peptides to increase his energy and rate of weight loss, as well as bioidentical testosterone to improve his sex drive.

The results? Joe lost twenty pounds in the process. After eighteen years of exercising and then increasing his intensity, he no longer has pain in his hips or legs—in other words, no claudication. He sleeps through the night and has more energy to do the activities he loves, from singing to spending active time with his grandkids.

Joe's story should encourage anyone that exercise is a powerful "drug" and can reverse many of the symptoms of the aging process. And it's never too late. At seventy-one, Joe is exercising harder and more vigorously than ever. And, he admits to feeling better today than he felt at age fifty-three.

An Anti-Aging Exercise Program

With each passing year, some of the things that can happen include loss of strength, diminished oxygen capacity, less flexibility, and impaired balance increasing the potential for falls. The good news is that you can prevent all of these from happening. The National Institute on Aging says, "When older people lose their ability to do things on their own, it doesn't happen just because they age. More likely it is because they have become inactive."

Rest assured that it is never too late to start exercising—no matter what your age. Exercise simply improves your quality of life while reversing aging. The best anti-aging exercises include those for strength, aerobic fitness, and flexibility. (Before you get started, especially if you've been inactive, get checked out by your doctor.)

If you have been sedentary up to this point, the best advice is to spend three to six months going for a walk for fifteen to forty minutes a day, five to seven days a week. If you can't walk, get an exercise bike and ride the exercise bike five to ten minutes twice a day. You can also try walking in water in a pool. It is helpful for your joints and a good way to move from sedentary to active.

Strength Training

There are numerous ways to improve strength. Many people are unfamiliar with going to the gym, and they don't understand the different ways to strength train. Today, a personal trainer can be extremely helpful in getting you started on a fitness regimen. You'll learn different ways to strengthen muscles, the importance of working muscle groups in order of importance—working large muscles first and then smaller ones to help maintain strength and balance—if you are working the whole body in one workout. In other words, you don't do triceps exercise before a bench press. Nor do you do biceps exercises before back exercises.

Another method is to work opposing muscle groups such as quadriceps (thighs) and hamstrings, biceps and triceps, chest and back, abs and lower back. So generally, strength training follows a pattern.

Understand the terminology, too. Repetitions, or reps, are the number of times you do an exercise. A set is the number of repetitions, and a superset usually represents working opposing muscle groups without rest.

Gym etiquette also is important; weights should always be returned to the rack or to weight holders after you complete your sets.

Weight workouts vary according to the level of experience. It is not uncommon to include dynamic exercises with static weight training, using dumbbells, barbells, and machines. A dynamic exercise would be pushups and pull-ups and the use of resistance bands; a static exercise would include machines that have pins in them, which are called selectorized machines; or free weights, which are usually barbells, dumbbells, and weight plates.

As a general rule, plates are usually 45, 35, 25, 10, and 5 pounds. A dumbbell rack starts at 5 pounds and can go up to 150-pound dumbbells. There are also multipurpose cable machines that can be utilized for varying body parts, flat, incline, and decline benches, as well as a barbell rack called a Smith machine that can be used at multiple heights.

There are varying routines that can improve strength. Most people who go to the gym go two to three times a week and work all muscle groups during a single workout. If that is your routine, the exercise order should be legs, back, chest, shoulders, biceps, and triceps. Because the abdominal muscles are a very small muscle group, they should be worked out almost daily with varying types of crunches, leg lifts, and abdominal machines.

A standard workout would be eight to ten repetitions with three sets for upper body; twelve to fifteen repetitions and three sets for the lower body. The number of exercises for each muscle group depends on the time you have.

Try to rest between sets. The rest interval is determined by whether you are trying to build strength or endurance in the muscles. For strength, a rest interval of ninety seconds is best. For endurance, it can be just thirty seconds.

If you are new to strength training, start with light weights or resistance bands and do each exercise for ten to fifteen reps. Use enough resistance (weight) that you can do the exercise no more than fifteen times. If you can do more, increase your weights. Progress by adding more weight, more reps, and more sets each week.

Let me add that you can also explore another form of strength training—bodyweight training—which requires little to no equipment. Instead, it relies on your body weight as the training modality, such as pushups and planks. This is a cost-effective way to get stronger without having to purchase expensive gym equipment.

Aerobic Exercise

To avoid heart disease, strokes, and vascular problems, you should always do aerobic activities, such as walking, jogging, swimming, rollerblading, and cycling, to name a few. Select the one(s) you enjoy and are most comfortable doing. Perform them at least thirty minutes three times a week.

There is a push now for everyone to get involved in HIIT (high intensity interval training). HIIT combines intervals of high-energy exercises, followed by short periods of active recovery. It has various benefits: It is time saving, it builds aerobic fitness, and it helps burn fat.

However, HIIT has potentially high injury rates, particularly in people over age forty. Statistics reveal that nearly 70 percent of participants suffer an injury within the first year.

I counsel all my patients who want to do HIIT to have an exercise evaluation done first. I also recommend that you start with a five-minute warmup on an exercise bike. Then keep the interval at thirty seconds, followed by a one-and-a-half-minute recovery. Repeat this sequence eight to ten times over twenty to thirty minutes. Finish with a two- to five-minute cooldown.

Once you can accomplish this comfortably, increase the interval time from thirty to forty-five seconds and the recovery time from a minute and a half to a minute and fifteen seconds. With more experience, up the intensity to a one-minute interval with a one-minute recovery, and eventually, a one-and-a-half-minute interval with a thirty-second recovery.

Most of you that are reading this book are not going to start doing HIIT. Gentle aerobic activity would be for you in the form of a fifteen- to thirty-minute walk or leisurely bike ride.

I rarely choose swimming as a good activity because it requires a lot of training to become a good swimmer. Most of you know how to ride a bike, and most humans can walk.

I realize for those that have restrictions other activities should be selected. For those of you who are limited with physical activity because of arthritis or other illnesses, I recommend water aerobics to get started in a class setting. As you progress in your aerobic training from your fifteen- to thirty-minute walk, instead of increasing the time of the walk, increase the pace of the walk to get additional benefits. The average person can walk three to four miles per hour, which is 110 to 130 strides per minute. If you are accustomed to walking as your only activity; increase your speed until you are walking four miles per hour. If you are under six feet tall, four mph is a fast pace; if you are over six feet, you should be able to walk 4.2 to 4.5 mph before you must begin to jog. A common exercise that I like to introduce to people is to walk a block, jog a block, walk a block, jog a block and repeat this until they can jog for thirty minutes at whatever pace they can go.

You could always use a bicycle, an Exercycle, or a rowing machine. All of these exercises can be performed to increase cardiovascular endurance. It is always better to incorporate both upper body and lower body, so using rowing machines, Nordic track, cross-country skiing, or aerodyne bicycles (a brand made by Schwinn) all have added benefits because they incorporate more muscle groups. We can certainly always do three to five aerobic days a week with one day of HIIT. Remember, combining aerobics and strength training is always going to be more beneficial than any other anti-aging program I could design.

Aerobics and Strength Combo

In 1983, I met a physician named Leonard Schwartz who had invented a workout method called "heavy hands exercise." Basically, you carry hand-held weights while walking or jogging. His premise was that upper body exercise is extremely important in improving cardiovascular fitness.

I wanted to see for myself, so I did an experiment. I gave each of the patients in our cardiac rehabilitation program hand-held weights to use while walking on a treadmill or walking outdoors. The weights were light—only two to five pounds. They could swing them a bit or just hold them steady.

I measured their fitness level both before and after and compared it to those who did not use hand-held weights. Much to my surprise, we improved their overall fitness levels by 25–30 percent over a course of three months in patients who utilized the hand-held weights.

As I further pursued this experiment, I realized that people with cardiovascular disease often suffer from heart attacks while using their upper bodies to shovel snow and other similar activities. I felt that the heavy hands method could help prevent these incidents, so I began to teach all my patients the value of weight training the upper body.

I feel that using weights while performing aerobic exercise is an effective time-saver since it builds cardiovascular strength and cardio fitness at the time. It is also a good calorie burner that can help you shed pounds. And because walking is a low-impact activity, there is no shock loading of joints, meaning that this form of exercise is suitable for people with foot, ankle, knee, or hip problems; exercisers who are heavy; or anyone who prefers a less jarring workout.

ASK DR. BOB: Can I lift weights if I have heart disease?

Yes! There's is no question that individuals who have heart disease should always do upper body strength training, especially. It is one of those areas of the body that frequently has been ignored in patients with heart disease.

Upper body strength and flexibility are extremely important because they represent 25 percent of the cardiac output. That's the amount of blood pumped out by the heart. It is also important for you to do some aerobic upper body activity such as rowing or working out on an upper body ergometer.

Flexibility Workouts

Flexibility exercises are the next vital component to an anti-aging exercise program. After the age of fifty, good flexibility helps you perform daily activities while avoiding injuries—including back injuries. And let's face it: the potential is high. Back pain is the major debilitating injury in this country, with knee and neck injuries running a close tie for second. Everyone wants to avoid such injuries because, in addition to the pain they cause, joint or back problems can keep you from doing the things you want to do, such as dancing, playing sports, exercising, making love, or doing just about anything you enjoy. Becoming more flexible also helps prevent falls.

You can choose from many types of flexibility exercises, and with all the variety, it's easy to find something you like. According to the American College of Sports Medicine (ACSM), adults should do flexibility exercises a minimum of two or three days each week to improve flexibility.

Here's a look at various types of flexibility work:

Static Stretching. This involves slowly stretching a muscle/tendon group and holding the position for a period of ten to thirty seconds. Static stretches help improve flexibility and range of motion (ROM), a measurement of the distance and direction a joint can move to its full potential.

There are two types of static stretching: active and passive. Active stretching involves stretching a muscle group by actively contracting one group of muscles in opposition to another group. You do not use external forces, such as a stretch band or other body part, to achieve the stretch. Usually these stretches are only held for ten to fifteen seconds.

Passive stretching requires some sort of external force in order to achieve the stretch (e.g., another person or a stretching device). With passive stretches, you rely on the external force to hold the body part being stretched in place. These stretches can be held ten to thirty seconds.

Yoga. There are many types of yoga being taught in the United States: Hatha yoga, Vinyasa, Bikram (hot yoga), Kripalu, and power yoga, among others. Each incorporates different techniques while using similar poses and groups of exercises called *asanas*. One of the most commonly incorporated asanas are Sun Salutations.

Yoga stretches and tones all the muscles and joints, exercising every part of your body. Yoga imparts not only remarkable physical benefits, but emotional and spiritual benefits as well. I believe it is especially valuable for people in high-stress jobs.

Research backs up yoga as an anti-aging activity. A study conducted in New Delhi in 2017 explored the impact of yoga and meditation on cellular aging in healthy participants. Ninety-six people were enrolled in the twelve-week study. Markers of aging were recorded at the beginning of the study and again after twelve weeks. The researchers discovered some amazing benefits as a result of yoga: telomeres lengthened, cortisol was balanced, oxidation was low, mood hormones were elevated, and anti-aging genes (sirtuins) increased. So, yoga for anti-aging? Absolutely!

In addition to anti-aging, I recommend yoga for everyone with high blood pressure, heart disease, cancer, arthritis, and especially for those with back problems.

Many gyms, community centers, and private studios have yoga classes for all different levels—so it is fairly easy to get started and make yoga a regular part of your fitness program.

Tai Chi. This ancient Chinese practice has a number of different forms and incorporates movement and flexibility. There are various types of tai chi, including Wu style, Chan style, and Yan style, all of which incorporate different movements.

In general, tai chi is a slow-moving process, based on defense mechanisms found in martial arts. Tai chi focuses on breathing and flowing gestures, which is why it is often called "meditation in motion." It exercises mind and spirit as well as body. And once you learn the basics, you can practice for as few as five minutes to as much as an hour a day. Just don't push yourself—the meditative effects of tai chi are important, too.

Several studies have found that tai chi exercises can help relieve pain, regulate blood pressure, build energy and strength, aid sleep, improve flexibility and balance, alleviate stress, and lessen the risk of falls. A 2004 study published in the *Archives of Physical Medicine and Rehabilitation* reported that tai chi also helped to slow bone loss in early postmenopausal women.

Additionally, arthritis sufferers are able to do tai chi because its low-impact movements place less stress on joints and muscles. A thirty-minute session twice a week for six months is enough to make a positive impact on your physical and emotional health.

Take lessons from a tai chi instructor who can make sure you're doing the movements correctly. Practice on your own after you've learned the basics and follow-up on corrections with the instructor.

To find a class in your community, contact the Arthritis Foundation (800–283–7800) or the Taoist Tai Chi Society at (850–224–5438/*www.taoist. org*). Your gym or local Y may also offer tai chi classes.

Pilates. This method of exercise was created in the 1920s by the physical trainer Joseph Pilates for the purpose of rehabilitation. Some of the first people treated by Pilates were dancers such as Martha Graham and George Balanchine, who wanted to strengthen their bodies and heal their aches and pains.

There are really two basic forms of Pilates: one utilizes a machine called the reformer; the other is a sequence of floor exercises that were originally designed by Joseph Pilates to teach people how to recover it by strengthening their core.

One of the basic differences between Pilates and yoga, other than the exercises, is that Pilates elongates, and yoga increases flexibility and strength. Also, Pilates works on core strengthening, which is a major component of rehabilitating from almost any injury of the back. Elongation of the spine and spaces between the vertebral bodies helps bring relief of chronic nerve pain—one of the strong benefits of Pilates. It also helps to increase the flexibility of all muscles inside the abdominal cavity known is the iliopsoas muscle. There are very few movements that will do this, other than Pilates.

Very recently, a patient named M. T. came to see me. He was a sixty-year-old man who had an injury at a very young age that not only hurt his back but also punctured a lung. Since his teenage years, he suffered with back pain brought on by minor motions like picking up a bar of soap in the shower. He walked tenuously for years because of this back pain, which greatly limited his golf game and many other activities.

After examining him, I found that he had one leg shorter than the other and inflexibility in his iliopsoas muscle and hamstrings.

I advised him that over the next year, he could improve these issues by using the reformer and Pilates exercises two to three days a week. After two months, I put him into a yoga class and had him do some basic strength-training moves. In only one month, M. T. had improved remarkably and was almost pain free with greater mobility. His case illustrates the power of flexibility exercises, along with some strength training.

ASK DR. BOB: Will exercising help me lose weight?

The best way to lose weight is to do repetitive exercises aerobically five to seven days a week and modify your nutrition. Exercise alone is not going to help you drop pounds if you don't change your diet. But it will increase your muscle mass—which is fat-burning, calorie-using tissue. The best way to lose weight is caloric restriction, intermittent fasting, or weekly fasting one day a week, along with a balanced exercise program.

Don't go overboard on exercising, however. Overdoing it might cause advanced aging because too much exercise increases free radicals and inflammation and shortens telomeres. You can tell you're overexercising if you're tired all the time, have constant muscle soreness, and get sick often.

Once you become more active, incorporating a variety of anti-aging exercises into your life, you'll find that the effort is more than worth it over time. With an active, fit body, you'll look more attractive, feel at your best, be able to do activities you did in your youth, and enjoy life even more.

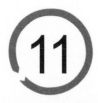

11

SEVEN NUTRITIONAL PITFALLS THAT PROMOTE AGING

If you want to stop "feeling your age," check *and correct* what you put in your mouth. The wrong foods, usually the processed and sugar-laden ones, are the source of oxidation and inflammation in the body—and they can definitely accelerate aging. If you are embracing the principles in this book, you must avoid these seven nutritional pitfalls.

Accelerated Ager 1:
Processed Foods

Many foods in the standard American diet hasten the aging process, and I'm talking about packaged foods, refined white flour and sugar, red meat, dairy products, fast food, most things that come in a box or package, and anything termed *junk food*. Processed foods are the arch enemies of youth because they:

Supply few nutrients. Your body requires at least thirty vitamins and minerals in order to function properly. The problem is that the body cannot make those raw materials on its own; they must be obtained from food, principally vegetables and fruits, and supplements. And yes, you do need supplements—unless you're living on an organic farm and eating organic foods that you grow and raise. So, take the supplements I recommend, and consider getting periodic vitamin infusions in order to shore up your body's anti-aging defenses.

Contain additives. These include added sugars, artificial sweeteners, and potentially dangerous substitutes, such as preservatives and colorings. All of these cause free-radical damage that accelerates aging and the incidence of many diseases, especially cancer. Artificially sweetened foods cause neurologic problems, loss of mental capacity, and poor fat metabolism.

Do a little experiment to test what I'm saying! Take a package of the pink, blue, or yellow artificial sweeteners and sprinkle them near an ant mound. Go back the next day and look at all the dead ants. Artificial sweeteners are all toxic to the nervous system. (Will the PETA people be protesting outside my office?)

Are loaded with pro-aging substances. These are trans fats, which promote inflammation and interfere with your ability to fight aging and genetically modified organisms (GMOs), which can promote weight gain and permanently alter the composition and function of the friendly bacteria in your gut.

Shorten telomeres. Using data from 840 adults from the Multi-Ethnic Study of Atherosclerosis, researchers found strong associations between nutrition and telomere length. Reporting in the *American Journal of Clinical Nutrition,* they noted that eating a lot of processed meats like bacon, sausage, luncheon meats, and ham could shorten your telomeres.

Telomeres are also shortened by obesity, which is partly the result of eating too many processed foods.

Are pro-inflammatory. In an eye-opening study published in the *Journal of the American College of Cardiology* in 2006, researchers pointed out that diets loaded with processed carbs, added sugar, saturated fats, and trans fats; and low in fruits, vegetables, whole grains, and omega-3 fatty acids are highly inflammatory. In contrast, though, a diet rich in whole foods, including natural, unprocessed carbohydrates, good fats, and lean protein sources, along with regular exercise and not smoking, counters inflammation.

Accelerated Ager 2:
Animal Foods

I rarely, if ever, eat animal foods—a dietary change that I began in February 1977. I had restarted my exercise program and was running several miles every day. But at five feet, ten inches, I weighed 240 pounds and obviously needed to trim down.

I had heard about vegetarian diets, which sounded healthy to me, so I decided to become a vegetarian for thirty days. This meant that I could still eat animal foods like cheese, milk, and eggs. At the same time, I increased my intake of vegetables and legumes.

During this "experiment" with my own body, I noticed that I was much more energetic than usual. I was losing weight. I felt great—so I decided to continue the diet for another thirty days.

Feeling even better, I slowly converted over to being a vegan. Vegans eat no animal products of any kind; it is a plant-based diet. I was at a meeting in Las Vegas at Caesar's Palace, ready to eat a meal, but as I looked at the menu, there was nothing that would fit a plant-based diet. I ordered stir-fried vegetables and moved the chicken to the side. A waitress came up to me and said, "What in the world are you doing?"

"I'm a vegetarian, and there is nothing on the menu for me to eat." I replied.

She smiled. "You're obviously a very stupid vegetarian. Why didn't you ask me for a vegetarian menu?"

I was in awe. The availability of plant-based menus solidified my intention of being a vegan for good.

By the end of 1977, I had lost approximately forty pounds, was running on a daily basis and training for my first marathon, and feeling that I had finally gotten a grasp on the value of plant-based nutrition. Over the last forty-two years, I've eaten some animal protein, but it always makes me feel sluggish, mentally and physically. I'm not going to try to convince you to become vegan, but I do emphasize the value of plant-based nutrition. It automatically removes the five aging pitfalls from your diet and is a game-changer in the world of anti-aging medicine.

In a breakthrough study by Marcia Martins in the journal *Nutrients* in 2017, 51,000 Seventh-Day Adventists (who are vegetarians) versus non-vegetarians were studied to determine the health outcome of their diets. The researchers reached three significant conclusions:

1. Non-vegetarians were more overweight and showed less healthy lifestyles than those who were either vegetarians or vegans.
2. Vegans who had practiced veganism most of their lives remained healthy well into their eighties.
3. Diets that reduce animal foods and adopt more vegetarian patterns have an anti-aging effect.

In another significant study, published in the *Harvard Newsletter* in 2018, researchers found that 76,000 vegetarians were on average 25 percent less likely to die of heart disease, compared to non-vegetarians.

The same *Harvard Newsletter* referenced a slew of studies suggesting that a diet with lots of fruits and vegetables can reduce the risk of developing certain cancers, and that vegetarians have a lower incidence of cancer then non-vegetarians. One of the cancers mentioned was colon cancer. Vegetarians usually have lower levels of potentially carcinogenic substances in their colons and consistently have lower cancer rates.

Other research has suggested that predominantly plant-based diets reduce the risk of type 2 diabetes by lowering BMI, weight, and total caloric intake.

I'm just scratching the surface here, but this growing mound of scientific evidence tells us that reducing or eliminating animal products in favor of more vegetables, fruit, grains, and legumes fights aging and the diseases of aging.

I cannot see a single health benefit to eating most animal proteins with the exception that you can easily increase the amount of protein in your diet. This helps preserve muscle mass, and it builds bulk. But it does not prolong your life span. This is a book about anti-aging, not bodybuilding.

Nonetheless, I also realize that a lot of people enjoy a good steak or chicken or fish. There are also people who hunt and enjoy wild game. Wild animals may be the healthiest animals you can eat because, unlike factory farm animals, they're not subjected to pollution, pesticides, hormones, and artificial diets. If you are going to eat animal protein, obviously wild game in the most pristine environment would be the best choice.

Bottom line: From my perspective, plant-based nutrition with limited exposure to animal protein is still the best way to reduce the incidence of chronic disease that has become so epidemic in our aging population.

Anti-Aging Pioneer: Dean Ornish, MD

Dean Ornish, MD, is a renowned cardiologist and best-selling author from California who conducted work with plant-based nutrition, meditation, and yoga on people who had been diagnosed with cardiovascular disease. He discovered that heart disease could be totally reversed with these methods. This was groundbreaking research that continues today, and still proves that lifestyle modification is the most effective treatment for cardiovascular disease.

Accelerated Ager 3:
Added Sugar

"Added sugar" means sugars and syrups added to foods. Desserts, candy, processed foods, and sodas are filled with added sugar. When you stir a tablespoonful of sugar into your coffee or tea, you are consuming added sugar.

If you eat a lot of foods with added sugar, the sugar can build up in your bloodstream. There, it attaches to proteins, hormones, and cells and produces advanced glycated end products (AGEs), which I discussed earlier. AGEs make your tissues stiffen and lose elasticity and can damage your eyes, kidneys, nerves, and other organs.

Added sugar thus ages you faster. It is also bad for health. When sugar is found in natural foods and plants (such as fruit), it comes packaged with all the vitamins, minerals, and enzymes needed for its complete digestion. But when it's sitting in your sugar bowl or added to your food, it has no nutritional value. Your body actually has to tap into its valuable storehouse of nutrients in order to process it. So, sugar literally robs your body of nutrients it otherwise really needs to stay healthy. For this reason, sugar is considered an immune system depressor. Added sugar is associated with obesity, diabetes, high blood pressure, and heart disease. It is also addictive.

Conventional nutritionists and physicians have suggested that it is okay to limit our consumption of sugar to five to six teaspoons in women and nine teaspoons in men. I disagree. It's just plain ridiculous to suggest that any amount of simple sugar is okay.

Accelerated Ager 4:
Gluten

Found mostly in wheat, rye, and barley, gluten is a protein that wears out your metabolism and immunity, making you appear older inside and out. By simply removing it from your diet plan, you can fight aging and allow your body to work naturally to maintain your vitality.

The number-one reason gluten ages you is that it produces oxidation. When gluten is oxidized in your body, the sulfur-containing amino acids it possesses build a network between the fibers and cause protein to harden. When this occurs, parts of the body (like your skin) lose their suppleness and elasticity, leading to pain and sagging skin.

In his bestseller *Grain Brain,* David Perlmutter, MD, describes the influence of gluten on increasing the incidence of neurologic diseases including Alzheimer's disease, dementia, Parkinson's, and ALS. I believe this is because gluten produces inflammation in the body.

For anti-aging (and not just treating celiac disease), adhere to a gluten-free diet.

Accelerated Ager 5:
Caloric Excess

We are in an evolutionary time in which a major problem in aging is that we eat too much food. We must cut back on the calories we eat daily if we want youth and vitality.

Fortunately, science shows that caloric restriction extends life in all animals, including humans. One of the ways you can easily achieve both caloric restriction and health is by becoming a vegan, according to the Physician's Committee, a group of medical doctors and nutritional savvy healers who have proven that plant-based nutrition slows aging and prevents disease. A plant-based diet automatically cuts calories, and you don't have to count them.

How does caloric restriction (CR) fight aging? It appears to help the body process insulin more normally (proper insulin regulation promotes anti-aging). Insulin fights being overweight and obesity—two situations that cause aging and shorten telomeres. And CR saves the energy-processing actions of the cells so that they repair themselves properly. Having adequate cell repair, and maintaining it, is associated with longevity.

We see these factors in action in the people of Okinawa. They suffer very few diseases of aging and have the largest number of centenarians in the world. Their diets are based on vegetables, grains, soy, fruits, fish, and seaweed. But they eat 20 percent fewer calories than the rest of Japan and 40 percent less than we do in the United States. The Okinawans are living proof that eating less means living longer!

In another example, the people who lived in Biosphere 2, a closed-system experiment in caloric intake was 30 percent lower than normal, experienced positive health changes: lower systolic and diastolic blood pressure, reduction in blood glucose, insulin, lower body temperature, and better-regulated thyroid hormone levels. These values persisted over eighteen months after the participants left the experiment, suggesting that calorie restriction could be a health-changing event.

Accelerated Ager 6:
Poor Cooking Methods

Foods cooked with high heat create advanced glycation end products, or AGEs, that accelerate aging. (So does added sugar.) AGEs generate lots of free radicals that damage cells and tissues, weakening your immunity, and causing chronic inflammation. They also contribute to hardening of the arteries, stiff joints, wrinkles, and other signs of aging. Cooking temperature makes a difference: A fried egg has ten times the AGEs of a scrambled egg, for example.

AGEs are also rampant in processed foods such as American cheese, fast food, and soft drinks, in part because they are manufactured using high heat. Eat too many of these foods, and higher-than-normal levels of AGEs build up in your tissues and accelerate the aging process from the inside out.

Grilled foods are also high in AGEs. It's better to lightly sauté vegetables and proteins in olive oil or bake them at low temperatures (like 350 degrees). Do *not* microwave them since it destroys all the nutrients in food. Use a slow cooker, Air Fryer, or Insta Pot to preserve nutrient density.

Accelerated Ager 7:
Food Storage Technology

I believe we are in trouble as a society because of one invention: the process of refrigeration. It has ruined our nutrition. The reason is that refrigerators keep foods for too long, and food loses its nutrient concentration by the day. Fortunately, we can get around this by eating locally sourced foods or fresh organic foods, without GMOs and preservatives or refrigeration whenever possible. You can also buy frozen certified organic produce because they are picked and frozen immediately, rather than several days later like conventional produce.

ASK DR. BOB: Is there any one "best" anti-aging food?

Every so often, news breaks that this food or that food makes you young, and everyone starts eating that one food. This is a big mistake. If you eat only blueberries, thinking they are the secret to youth and long life, for example, you will miss out on many other nutrients in many other foods. Here's my take on this: there is no such thing as one magic food to cure aging. Human physiology is complex, and it takes multiple nutrients working together on a molecular level to get to the point in which your health and body begin to defy aging.

Following a dietary pattern as a whole is important, not just the individual components. This has been proven in studies of plant-based diets—characterized by frequent intake of fruits, vegetables, nuts, beans, whole grains, and olive oil—and shown to slow aging. This eating pattern has been shown to prevent telomere shortening, and the suspected reason is that it is rich in omega 3 fatty acids, vitamins, antioxidants and fiber, and void of regular consumption of less-healthy foods that speed up aging. The bottom line is that it's not the single anti-aging foods you eat, but a sum of its parts that is key.

Finally, Avoid the "Square Pig"

Every grocery store in this country is designed to lure you into the center of the store, where all the processed foods are stacked, while the fresh foods are on the periphery of the store. I call the center of every supermarket "the square pig." Other than paper goods or soap, there is no food in this area of the market that you cannot live without.

More specifically, you will walk right into the bakery as soon as you enter the store. And there may be flowers there to further entice you. Stop—and stay on the periphery, where you will first find fruits, vegetables, nuts, and seeds.

Located on the very edge of the square will usually be fish, poultry, meat, and dairy items, including cheeses.

The store usually puts wine, drinks, organic chips, and other so-called pseudo-foods there to lure you to enter the square pig. But if you stay on the edges of the store, you'll find everything you need for anti-aging and great health.

Just know that there is a marketing madness to the method to get you to buy unhealthy stuff—and basically make bad choices. But if you avoid these choices and the processed foods that accelerate aging, you will avoid obesity, diabetes, heart disease, and other scary conditions that make you old before your time.

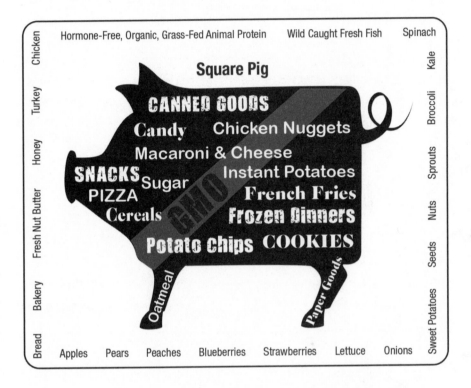

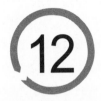

Solution:

REJUVENATION NUTRITION

Very recently, I ran into a friend of mine at a local pizzeria. He is in his forties, extremely healthy looking, and very fit. He was eating a large, white-bread garlic roll.

"That looks good," I commented.

"I can eat anything I want because I work out and never gain an ounce," he replied.

As we walked away, I said to my wife, "Let him tell me that when he is sixty and has a stroke or a heart attack."

If such a tragedy were to happen to this guy, most people would be shocked. But when it comes to aging, nutrition is truly the gold standard in fighting it. In medicine, when we use the term "gold standard," we are describing a method or procedure that is regarded as the best available. So it is with nutrition—the gold standard in anti-aging measures. If you're not feeding yourself with the essential nutrients, your body will age faster.

And that's regardless of how active or athletic you are. Take the example of Jim Fixx, a well-known runner and author in the '80s. Fixx knew he had high cholesterol and a family history of heart disease, yet he ignored the warning signs.

One day while on a run, he noticed that his pace had lessened. Jim was often able to run ten miles in sixty minutes or less as a training run. Suddenly he realized this pace slowed, first to eight-minute miles and then to nine- or ten-minute miles, and yet he continued to enjoy his runs. One day, after completing a run and waiting to cross the road, he collapsed and died of a massive heart attack.

This story is pertinent to aging and age-related diseases because many people think exercise is the key. It's not. Although exercise is important, good nutrition trumps exercise every time.

So, let's pick up the subject of nutrition—and how to eat to reverse and prevent aging.

The Rejuvenation Solution Eating Plan

You'll kick this plan off with my 7-day program in chapter 15, but it is a plan you'll want to stick with for a long life. Over the course of the past ten years, every single one of my patients who has followed the Rejuvenation Solution Eating Plan has experienced the following: more energy, a reduction in heart disease markers (LDL cholesterol, total cholesterol, blood pressure, and an increase in HDL), weight loss and lower body fat levels, better blood sugar control, hormone balance (often in conjunction with bioidentical hormone replacement), reduced inflammation, and an outward glow. These are all signs that aging has slowed down in their bodies.

The patients who achieved these benefits followed my plan for ninety days, and continued it beyond ninety days with some modifications. This is what I recommend that you do as well.

First, here's what you won't eat—and why—on the plan.

Simple Starches and Sugars

Absolutely no rice, potatoes, pasta, white flour, or products made from these foods. This includes most packaged cereals as well. Potato chips, cookies, pancakes, pastry, and crackers are on the forbidden list, too. No sweetened foods either—no candy, syrups, jellies, or jams. Refined sugar is one of the most damaging and aging substances we can put into our bodies. To me, it's a dangerous drug that causes skin wrinkling and organ damage—not to mention mood swings, depression, and energy crashes.

Bread

At least try to go without bread for ninety days. You can obtain the fiber in bread from fruits and vegetables. Once you eliminate sandwiches from your diet, you will automatically become healthier. If you miss a food you can hold in your hand like a sandwich, try rolling your lunch foods in a large lettuce or collard green leaf like a tortilla.

Alcohol, Caffeine, and Artificial Sweeteners

All three of these substances generate free radicals and thus stimulate cell degeneration. They also interfere with fat metabolism. If you have to sweeten something, use the herb stevia.

Foods with Preservatives

These foods—which are generally found in packages and boxes—cause free-radical damage that has almost certainly increased the incidence of many diseases, including, most importantly, cancer. We were meant to eat freshly prepared foods.

Most Condiments

Most salad dressings and ketchup contain high amounts of sugar, and mayonnaise has too much fat. Keep away from these bottled non-foods. Healthier choices include:

Herbs and spices
Homemade salad dressings made with olive oil and vinegar
Mustards
Horseradish
Natural ketchup (no sugar added)
Sriracha
Soy sauce (low sodium)
Frank's Wing Sauce
Salsa
Hot sauce
Vinegars

Certain High-Sugar Vegetables and Fruits

These include beets, corn, bananas, mangoes, and grapes. Although these foods are packed with nutrients as well as carbohydrates, they do fall in the category of high-sugar foods, and they tend to spike your blood sugar quickly. So, you'll need to forego them for ninety days and return them to your diet in moderate amounts afterward.

What You Can and Should Eat

Right about now, you might be asking, "If you tell me to eliminate all those foods, what is left?"

Food is medicine, and the right food is anti-aging. And your body's best defense against aging and disease is food that fights oxidation, inflammation, telomere shortening, and other causes of aging. Here are the foods that will accomplish that.

Plant Foods

A very recent piece of research, published in the journal *Current Opinion in Clinical Nutrition and Metabolic Care*, stated something that I have been advocating for years, and discussed in the previous chapter, that plant-based diet, including five daily helpings of fruits and vegetables (two fruits and three to five vegetables), is a key mainstay of aging successfully.

I recommend that you omit animal products from your diet for at least thirty days and see how you look and feel. If you like your results, continue a plant-based diet for another thirty days or longer.

Why does plant-based nutrition slow the aging clock?

There are four cellular events at work:

Antioxidants. To stay young, forget about carbohydrates, protein, and fat, and instead focus on fruits, vegetables, nuts, and seeds. As a source of antioxidants, these foods wipe out oxidative stress responsible for aging the body and promoting diseases of aging. There's plenty of proof of just how powerfully nutrition like this can fight aging.

Telomerase Activity. When your body turns telomerase on, you start to make long telomeres of your DNA. There are foods now known clinically to increase telomerase activity. Legumes are one of them. They're high in plant chemicals called isoflavones, which stimulate telomerase and thus delay the aging of the cells, and they are rich sources of the B vitamin, folic acid, which plays an important role in DNA integrity and repair (both of which decline with age). Nuts count, too. They're loaded with omega-3 fatty acids and vitamin E, two nutrients that have a positive influence on telomerase. Eating any antioxidant-rich, plant-derived food helps maintain telomere length.

Anti-Inflammatory Action. The same plant-based diet that supplies antioxidants and stimulates telomerase also quenches inflammation in the body. As long as you eat the right foods—with an emphasis on plant foods—your body is powerfully equipped to make its own anti-inflammatory compounds. Such a diet slashes your risk of chronic diseases associated with aging, such as heart disease, diabetes, cancer, and neurodegenerative diseases.

The Top Eight Anti-Inflammatory Foods

1. Kale

This green leafy veggie is loaded with anti-inflammatory phytonutrients and antioxidants that help protect our bodies against cellular damage. It is also a great source of amino acids; vitamins A, C, and K; fiber; and the minerals magnesium, iron, and calcium. Its anti-aging benefits include more youthful skin, healthy eyes, great digestion, and strong bones. Add kale to your salads and smoothies.

2. Pineapple

Although a high-glycemic fruit (it contains a lot of natural sugar), it packs a big punch! It is loaded with vitamin C and contains a special enzyme called bromelain that may help stimulate protein digestion, reduce inflammation of the gut, and boost immune function. Eat it raw or add it to smoothies.

3. Wild Salmon

This cold-water fish is the only animal food I recommend because it is one of the best sources of omega-3 fatty acids, which fight inflammation, lower risk for chronic diseases, and improve mental health. Salmon is also high in protein and rich in vitamins B12, B3, D, and the minerals potassium and selenium.

4. Mushrooms

Mushrooms are powerhouses because they contain compounds called beta-glucans that help to improve immunity and lower inflammation throughout the body. There is also a potent antioxidant in mushrooms called ergothioneine that fights inflammation. Mushrooms are rich in protein, fiber, and various B vitamins, too. Some of my favorite varieties are shiitake, morel, chanterelle, and porcini mushrooms.

5. Broccoli

Packed with vitamins C and K, folate, and fiber, broccoli is an anti-inflammatory treasure trove. It's especially rich in antioxidants like the flavonoids kaempferol and quercetin, as well as a variety of carotenoids. Sauté this veggie up with garlic, onion, and shiitake mushrooms for a delicious anti-inflammatory dish.

6. Dulse

Dulse is a type of seaweed rich in compounds called fucoidans, which reduce inflammation within the body. This unique sea vegetable is also packed with iron, potassium, iodine, fiber, and proteins. You can eat dulse fresh or dried. Try adding it to green leafy salads, chopped up with avocado, or blended into dressings.

7. Blueberries

Low in sugar and high in fiber, blueberries are full of vitamins A, C, and E, and contain a variety of anti-inflammatory properties and antioxidants.

The major antioxidant, anthocyanin, is what gives this berry its deep blue color. Eat blueberries as a snack or add them to cereal or yogurt.

8. Sauerkraut/Kimchi

Also known as fermented cabbage, sauerkraut contains probiotics to help tame inflammation in the gut. It is also rich in vitamins C and K, iron, and fiber. Kimchi is a Korean staple that includes napa cabbage and other fermented vegetables. Try adding sauerkraut and kimchi to your green salads or on top of veggie burgers.

Bioenergetics. This term refers to the production and transformation of energy in cells. When you eat food, it is converted into chemical energy that your body absorbs and stores as glycogen, fat, and protein. Then, when needed, it is released to provide energy to produce adenosine triphosphate (more commonly known at ATP), a high-energy molecule for muscular contractions and a variety of other metabolic and life-sustaining functions in your body.

More than 95 percent of the ATP produced in the body occurs in the mitochondria, the energy factories of cells. The nutrient coenzyme Q10 (CoQ10) is a critical cofactor in the production of ATP.

Unfortunately, CoQ10 levels continuously decrease as we age, resulting in a cascade of negative events, including cardiovascular disease, neurodegenerative disease, and skin wrinkling. One of the many ways to resist aging, then, is to make sure you supply your body with ample CoQ10. The best food sources of this nutrient are plant-based foods. In fact, vegetarians usually have twice of the levels of this nutrient in their bodies than meat-eaters do. This indicates that a high level of plant foods may help preserve, even boost, CoQ10 levels.

Another advantage of plant-based eating is that it automatically lowers your caloric intake, and you don't have to count calories. This is important because calorie restriction is a bona fide anti-ager.

Remember the Okinawans? A study published in December 2003 in *Science of Aging Knowledge Environment* shows that older Okinawans who consumed the traditional plant-based diet did not gain weight with age.

This finding supports the caloric restriction findings of previous studies that show that low calorie intake can increase your life span by up to 50 percent. The key is to reduce your caloric intake by about 30 percent. You can do this by eating more plant foods and water-rich foods such as veggie soups, and by eating more fiber such as vegetables.

Go Raw

It's not enough to emphasize plant foods; it's just as important to eat at least 80 percent of these foods in their raw state. Raw foods include fruits, vegetables, nuts, sprouts, and seeds prepared in a way that maintains the food's enzymes and other nutrients. Cooking food can deplete many essential minerals, most vitamins, and all of the enzymes. It also interferes with the bioelectrical energy necessary to sustain life; literally, the life force is cooked out of food.

In terms of anti-aging, raw food:

- Enhances the functioning capacity of digestive enzymes. As we age, our natural digestive enzymes are depleted, allowing food to ferment (rot) in the digestive tract. I concur with the many experts who believe that this undigested matter becomes quite toxic, causing many of the health problems associated with aging;
- Delivers oxygen to the organs and tissues;
- Detoxifies the body, mainly through the intake of chlorophyll from green, leafy vegetables;
- Supplies vital nutrients to the endocrine and nervous system (sprouted seeds and legumes are particularly powerful at this);
- Supports and sustains weight loss—without the need to count calories, carbohydrates, fats, and so forth.
- Prevents cardiovascular disease, the leading cause of death in the US. Research into raw foods has shown that they favorably modify a gene called 9p21—the strongest genetic marker for heart disease.

Plant Proteins

You'll need protein to build and maintain lean muscle mass—and to repair tissue. You can obtain your protein from the following plant sources:

Beans and legumes.

Nuts and seeds, including sprouted seeds and legumes.

Nut milks such as almond milk, cashew milk, coconut milk, and hemp milk.

Nondairy yogurt, such as that made from almond milk.

Cereals and grains. Grains like quinoa, barley, and oats are high in protein.

Lacto-ovo vegetarian proteins. If you want to gradually cut down on meat, it's fine to eat cheese (in moderation) and eggs. This is one approach to vegetarianism.

Also, if you do not want to cut out animal protein entirely, eating fish twice a week is fine (this is the pesco-vegetarian approach to eating). But avoid bottom-feeder fish, such as shellfish, grouper, catfish, and flounder. They eat things that have died from unnatural causes and may contain toxins. Better choices are wild sources of tuna, mackerel, salmon, and trout.

Ten Veggies with the Most Protein

One of the misconceptions of plant-based nutrition is that you can't get all the protein you need from plant foods. Nothing could be further from the truth. Plant foods are loaded with protein—plus anti-aging, anti-inflammatory antioxidants that enhance quality of life and longevity. Other than protein from beans, legumes, nuts, and seeds, here's a list of plant foods that also pack a lot of protein.

1. Watercress

Grown in water, watercress contains 0.8 grams of protein in one cup. Protein accounts for 50 percent of its calories. Eat watercress raw because cooking it destroys its high antioxidant content. It tastes great in salads and on sandwiches.

2. Sprouts

Sprouts referred to a number of vegetable or plant beans after they begin to grow. I grow my own sprouts occasionally but often purchase it from an organic reputable sprouting firm called *gotsprouts.com*. I find the addition of sprouts increases my available protein and obviously an incredible amount of minerals and vitamins and enzymes that I can't always get from fresh organic vegetables that are grown locally. One cup (33 grams) of alfalfa sprouts, for example, provides 1.3 grams of protein; protein accounts for 42 percent of its calories.

My favorite salad is a combination of cabbage, spinach, kale, zucchini, cucumber, radishes, avocado, snow peas, chickpeas, onion, tomato, and three or four different types of sprouts.

Red flag: Raw sprouts (the best way to eat them) have been linked to outbreaks of foodborne illnesses like *E. coli* and other potentially serious infections. Purchase sprouts only from reputable sources and wash them thoroughly before serving.

3. Spinach

Spinach is a superfood. Protein makes up about 30 percent of its calories, and it contains all the essential amino acids. A one-cup serving provides 1 gram of protein. Besides its high protein content, spinach is full of plant compounds that can increase antioxidant defense and reduce inflammation.

4. Chinese cabbage

Also known as bok choy, Chinese cabbage is another tasty source of vegetable protein. One cup (70 grams) of Chinese cabbage contains 1 gram of protein. Chinese cabbage accentuates Asian recipes, such as stir-fries, kimchi, soups, and spring rolls.

5. Asparagus

A one-cup serving of asparagus contains 2.9 grams of protein. It is also a powerful prebiotic, anti-inflammatory, and anti-cancer food. You can roast asparagus in the oven, or grill, boil, steam, or pan-fry it.

6. Mustard greens

Very similar to kale but with a distinct mustard flavor, mustard greens provide 1.5 grams of protein in a single serving (1 cup). Protein accounts for 25 percent of the calories in mustard greens. This veggie can be steamed, boiled, sautéed, or simply eaten raw in salads.

7. Broccoli

Broccoli is a very popular vegetable that also happens to be high in protein. A one-cup (91-gram) serving of raw chopped broccoli supplies 2.6 grams of protein, including all the essential amino acids. Broccoli has anti-cancer, anti-cholesterol, and detoxification properties. It can be enjoyed raw or cooked. You can use it to make tasty side dishes, soups, and sauces.

8. Collard greens

Collard greens are a delicious, dark green, large-leafed vegetable. A one-cup serving contains 0.9 grams of protein. Collard greens can be steamed or sautéed. They are tasty when cooked with onions and mushrooms. You can also use the large leaves to make breadless sandwich wraps.

9. Brussels sprouts

A one-cup (88-gram) serving of Brussels sprouts contains 3 grams of protein. Protein accounts for 19 percent of the calories in this food. You can cook Brussels sprouts by boiling, steaming, grilling or roasting. They are an ideal side dish.

10. Cauliflower

Like broccoli, cauliflower provides a high amount of protein. One cup (100 grams) of cauliflower has 2 grams of protein. Protein accounts for 19 percent of its calories. Cauliflower has become very popular as a substitute for potatoes and other starchy carbs. You can enjoy it raw, baked, or mashed.

Fats

Fats are essential to your diet because they contain vitamins, such as A, D, E, and K. Plus, they are required to form hormones in the body. Good choices include:

Avocadoes

Avocado oil

Olives

Olive oil

Coconut oil

Nut oils (almond and walnut oils)

Sesame oil

Tahini

Nut butters

No doubt you're aware of the importance of eating omega-3 fatty acids, which are abundant in oily fish like tuna, mackerel, and salmon. Omega-3s are key for heart and brain health, joint mobility, cancer protection, and many other aspects of health. But did you know that you can obtain these vital fats from plant foods?

That's right. Good plant sources of omega-3s are chia seeds, Brussels sprouts, algal oil, hemp seeds, walnuts, and flaxseeds.

ASK DR. BOB: What if I don't like vegetables?

I often get asked this question, and it's usually from people who were not raised with vegetables in their diets as kids. That's sad because they've missed out on a food group that reduces oxidative stress and inflammation and stops the shortening of telomeres and improves hormone balance.

If you're in the "I don't like vegetables" camp, I suggest at least trying to find some veggies (and fruits) that you do like. Then try "sneaking" veggies into other foods, such as soups, stews, casseroles, smoothies, and on top of pizza.

Taste for foods is something you can acquire. Eat veggies like this consistently, and eventually you'll develop a taste for them.

Your Anti-Aging Eating Routine

Here's a look at how you can structure your day to incorporate my anti-aging food strategies.

Breakfast

Start your day with fruit—half of a grapefruit, fourth of a melon, a cup of berries, a pear, an apple, or a peach. Serve it with a half-cup to cup of oatmeal, topped with chopped almonds, and some nut milk. Or you might make yourself an omelet with two eggs, plus some spinach and feta cheese. Another option is to make a breakfast smoothie with nut milk, frozen unsweetened berries, and a handful of raw spinach or kale. For your beverage, choose hot water and lemon or herbal tea.

Mid-Morning Snack

A serving of fruit (but remember to avoid bananas and mangoes for thirty to ninety days). Or, have a smoothie like the one suggested for breakfast.

Lunch

Have at least six ounces of a vegetable protein such as beans, legumes, or lentils; a vegetable burger; lentil or split pea soup, or vegetable soup. Alternatively, have a large mixed green salad with lots of raw veggies topped with legumes, cheese, or chopped eggs. Add some nuts or seeds to the salad or even a fourth of an avocado. Dress the salad with balsamic vinegar mixed with one of the vegetable oils listed previously. Try to have at least one raw salad daily.

Afternoon Snack

A serving of fruit (but remember to avoid bananas and mangoes for ninety days). Or, have cut-up raw vegetables dipped in hummus.

Dinner

At least six ounces of vegetable protein with two cooked vegetables of different colors—for example, summer squash and okra, or asparagus and cauliflower. Have a tossed salad of raw veggies, similar to the one you had at lunch. Or enjoy a vegetarian soup and salad, or a cauliflower vegetable pizza and salad.

Beyond the Ninety Days

Introduce foods back into your diet that were completely eliminated the first ninety days, such as beets, corn, bananas, grapes, and mangoes.

You can also add some starchy foods back into your diet, but eat them in moderation. Restrict potatoes to no more than one or two a week, and choose mostly sweet potatoes or yams in preference to white potatoes. Eliminate white rice altogether and eat brown rice or basmati, a whole-grain white rice. Restrict rice to no more than three times a week. If you must eat pasta, make sure it is made from vegetable sources (like chick peas or black beans) or is a whole-grain pasta. Try mixing these pasta with zoodles (strands of zucchini that sub for regular pasta) or fettuccine made from butternut squash. Make sure the bread you eat is rye, whole-grain, or sprouted. Ideally, eat them only at breakfast.

Drink no more than two or three glasses of wine a week, or one drink of distilled liquor per week. And stay away from beer! It promotes fat production. Drinking alcoholic beverages produces sugar cravings, so it's best to stay away from them.

Ideally, eat three main meals daily—but not the huge meals in the typical American style. I recommend that you follow the lead of other cultures that have maintained good health, sound nutrition, and longevity and eat a light breakfast. Then eat your main meal prior to 2 PM Finish with a light evening meal, and if possible, don't eat anything after 7 PM.

The important thing is that you make informed choices—that you stop blindly putting food and drink into your body without paying attention to foods that affect your health and rate of aging.

ASK DR. BOB: Is the keto diet a good diet for anti-aging?

No! First, some background: A keto diet severely limits carbohydrates to under 20 grams a day (no fruits, except maybe some occasional berries) and increases fat from animals and plants to 75 percent of your total daily calories. The idea is to put your body into "ketosis," a state of fat-burning.

There are a couple of big problems with this type of eating plan. When you restrict carbohydrates so much, you're missing out on a lot of anti-aging antioxidants, in fruits, especially. Also, animal protein is allowed, and I have just established that eating plants over animals is superior to fight aging. Finally, the high-fat nature of the keto diet is highly inflammatory, and inflammation is at the root of most diseases and a significant driver of aging. Please know that there are numerous studies that suggest that being in ketosis for a prolonged period of time shortens life span.

A study published in *Lancet Public Health* looked at low-carb diets like the keto diet in more than 15,000 people over age twenty-five and followed them for twenty-five years. The researchers concluded that a keto diet shortens life span by almost four years. Further, when the American Heart Association looked at low-carbohydrate, high-animal-protein diets, it found that there was a 43 percent increase in heart failure. If the source of animal protein came from dairy, it increased the risk of heart failure to 49 percent.

So basically: the data says that the ketone diet may be not only shortening life span, but it also increases overall cardiovascular risk. I am vehemently opposed to a ketogenic diet for these reasons.

13

Cause 7:

STRESS

There's no doubt that chronic stress accelerates aging.
Just look at how much older presidents of the United States appear
after eight years in one of the most stressful jobs that anyone can have.
Stress is the silent killer and the silent ager. It does its damage largely by
promoting inflammation in chromosomal processes, including telomere
length, leading to disease.

The effects of too much stress wreak havoc on the brain and, indeed,
the entire body. Physicians and scientists who study the connections
between psychology, neurology, the endocrine system, and the nervous
system have shown that thoughts and emotions—typically triggered
by physical, emotional, or environmental stressors—create chemical
changes in the brain. I believe these chemical changes, whether caused
by an emotion, virus, or a carcinogen, are a chief cause of aging and disease. They can change cell chemistry in such a way that the cell's DNA
receives a message to alter the way in which the cell functions. Cancer
may begin as this cellular level, for example, or diabetes may occur.

When too many stimuli from the outside world bombard your central nervous system (the brain, spinal cord, and associated nerve endings), the result is an imbalance. This imbalance might manifest itself as symptoms of overactivity: your mind races, you have insomnia, and you can't relax. Eventually, your stomach, heart, and skin are affected. You might develop digestive diseases, such as Crohn's disease, irritable bowel syndrome, or chronic constipation.

Such overstimulation can also trigger the opposite effect: you're always tired, you sleep too much, and you can't concentrate. Eventually, this can lead to chronic fatigue syndrome, slow circulation to the heart and other organs, platelet stickiness, and heart attacks and heart disease.

The Nervous System: Relax or Respond?

The body's nervous system is divided into two parts, designed to help you deal with and adapt to short-term, immediate stress: the sympathetic nervous system (SNS) and the parasympathetic nervous system (PNS). They balance each other out.

The SNS mobilizes your body's resources for "fight or flight" in threatening situations. The PNS helps the body rest, recover, and seek peace. In the PNS state, cells require less oxygen, they store energy more efficiently, and they repair DNA in the mitochondria. The PNS state also improves blood flow throughout the body for organ repair, while protecting the brain from the excess cortisol produced by chronic stress. The body is designed to spend the majority of its time in the PNS, while activation of the SNS is reserved for true life-threatening emergencies.

Our hectic lives trigger the SNS. So do worry and mental stress because the body cannot differentiate between a real or imagined stress. Thus, if you constantly worry and think about stressors, such as being late on bills, rehashing an argument at home, or experiencing job problems, the SNS is activated through your imagination alone.

Recovery from stress requires techniques to reduce the dominance of the SNS and to activate PNS. With the PNS activated, your body begins to repair and restore from damage caused by stress—and healing begins. This is called putting the body in a "parasympathetic repair state" (and it is something our prevailing medical system ignores). It can be accomplished by exercise, relaxation exercises, quality sleep, meditation, hypnosis, and other restorative methods. We can and will improve our physical health when we take care of our parasympathetic nervous system. The next chapter will give you the solutions to healing from within.

What Is Stress Doing to Your Health?

It has been estimated that more than 85 percent of all visits to doctors' offices are for stress-related disorders. Why is this? Because stress does promote illness; there's no question about it. In short, a stressor provokes a reaction from the central nervous system, and the adrenal glands almost instantly—the so-called fight or flight response. The immediate response is a fast heart rate, sweaty palms, a rise in blood pressure, an increase in production of acid in the stomach, and an outpouring of inflammatory chemicals called cytokines.

As a society, we must learn that too many hours of work, too few hours of sleep, too many pro-inflammatory foods, too many electronic devices, and other stressors are depleting antioxidants, decreasing telomerase, shortening telomeres, increasing inflammation, and interfering with the normal function of hormones. The compounding effect is vulnerability to serious disease. Parkinson's, ALS, depression, Alzheimer's, hostility and anger, and suicide rates are signs of a deteriorating health care model that could destroy the world as we know it. We are a society that is increasing our life span but also increasing our *sick span*.

In 1967, psychiatrists Thomas Holmes and Richard Rahe analyzed the medical records of more than 5,000 medical patients in order to prove whether stressful events might indeed cause illness. Patients checked off events from a list of forty-three life events called Life Change Units (LCUs); their answers were scored.

Holmes and Rahe were able to correlate associations between their life events and their illnesses. The results were published as the Social Readjustment Rating Scale (SRRS), known more commonly as the Holmes and Rahe Stress Scale. It also emphasized that the effects of various types of psychosocial stressors are additive. Subsequent validation has supported the links between stress and illness.

I've adapted the scale a bit. To assess how stressed you might be, and if you are at risk for illness, please take the following assessment. Circle the events that have occurred in your life over the last twelve to eighteen months and add up the life change units (LCUs) that correspond with each one.

1. Death of spouse → 100

2. Divorce → 73

3. Marital separation → 65

4. Jail term → 63

5. Death of a close family member → 63

6. Personal injury or illness → 53

7. Marriage → 50

8. Fired from job → 47

9. Physical, emotional, sexual abuse → 45

10. Retirement → 45

11. Change in health of a family member → 44

12. Pregnancy → 40

13. Sex difficulties → 39

14. Gaining a new family member → 39

15. Business readjustment → 39

16. Change in financial state → 38

17. Death of a close friend → 37

18. Change to a different line of work → 36

19. Reduction in energy level, more fatigue → 35

20. Mortgage/loan for major purchase (home, etc.) → 31

21. Foreclosure of mortgage or loan → 30

22. Change in responsibilities at work → 29

23. Rarely laugh → 29

24. Trouble with in-laws → 29

25. Outstanding personal achievement → 28

26. Spouse begins or stops work → 6

27. Twenty or more pounds overweight → 26

28. Change in living conditions → 25

29. Alcohol/recreational drug use five to seven times weekly → 24

30. Smoking → 23

31. Change in work hours or conditions → 20

32. Change in residence → 20

33. Change in schools → 20

34. Change in recreation → 19

35. Change in church activities → 19

36. Change in social activities → 19

37. Mortgage/loan for lesser purchase (car, etc.) → 17

38. Change in sleeping habits → 16

39. Sedentary lifestyle → 15

40. Change in eating habits to more junk food → 15

41. Feeling depressed or anxious a lot → 13

42. Have few friends → 12

43. Minor violations of the law → 11

Results:

0–150 LCUs: Your level of stress is low, and your risk of disease is low.

150–300 LCUs: Borderline stress level. You should attempt to minimize changes in your life at this time. Your risk of illness could be as high as 50 percent.

More than 300 LCUs: Your stress levels are high. Your risk of disease could be as high as 80 percent. You should minimize changes in your life and institute some stress intervention techniques.

Adapted from: Rahe, R.H., and Arthur, R.J. 1978. Life change and illness studies: Past history and future directions. Journal of Human Stress 4: 3–15.

The Upside of Stress

On a positive note, we need some stress in order to survive. It gives us an edge in times of danger. It's what helped our ancestors survive their encounters with saber-toothed tigers. Levels of the stress hormone cortisol soared to energize them to deal with the danger and then returned to normal after it was over. So, when our ancestors encountered threats to their survival, it was often short lived.

The same reaction kicks in today as we deal with modern stressors. Our adrenal glands pump out the hormones cortisol, epinephrine, and norepinephrine, triggering the sympathetic and parasympathetic nervous systems to raise blood pressure, increase heart rate, and cause other physical changes.

Cortisol, when released in short spurts by the adrenals, acts as an anti-inflammatory agent. It helps rally glucose and fatty acids in the body in order to produce energy and nourish tissues.

The adrenals also start producing adrenaline. This hormone makes your heart beat faster and harder and elevates your blood pressure to help you respond to the stressor.

Next, the hormones of the brain, including serotonin, dopamine and other neurotransmitters, signal your nerves to react—so that you have a heightened sense of danger and can respond. What's more, your liver starts to pump out cholesterol to provide your body with fuel.

This cascade of physiological events helps your body prepare to take action and can be lifesaving.

When Stress Is Chronic

When we are exposed to chronic stress, such as the emotional demands of work deadlines, verbal reprimands or abuse, negative thinking, radiation from cell phones and dental x-rays, money worries, raising kids, and countless other stressors, our cortisol levels tend to rise and to remain elevated longer than normal. These types of stressors are "the saber-toothed tigers" of our time. One problem is that most of these are there every day, and therefore, chronic levels of the adrenal hormone cortisol cause high blood pressure, obesity, heart disease, inflammation of the brain, and eventually organ failure of the adrenals themselves.

The cortisol mechanism is scary because when it stays elevated in the body, this can lead to brain fog, Alzheimer's, neurotoxicity, heart failure, and death.

Chronic stress has an effect on all the other causes of aging and may indeed be the least understood and also the most neglected part of medicine. Stress causes all the hormones to wear out faster, thereby causing lower testosterone, higher insulin and cortisol, and lower melatonin levels. The result is reduced energy, poor sleep, increased body weight, and decline in muscle mass.

Unresolved stress shortens telomeres, too. For instance, among twenty- to fifty-year-old mothers who had been caring for a chronically ill child, telomere length was related to the duration of caregiving; the longer the caregiving, the shorter the telomeres are. This finding supports the notion that too much stress is bad for the body, and that it contributes to the wear-and-tear, which results in aging.

Stress and Your Gut

Think about the last time you felt stressed out. Did your stomach clench up in knots or did you feel butterflies? What was going on, exactly?

Stress has a big impact on your gut. Your gut can send stress messages to your brain and vice versa. A troubled gut can signal the brain, just as a troubled brain can signal the gut. The connection goes both ways.

The gut is regulated by the enteric nervous system (ENS), a complex system of about 100 million nerves that originates in the brain and ends in the gut. It controls the entire digestive process, so it's not surprising that when you get upset, your gut gets upset. The nerve endings of the ENS transmit messages from the brain to the gut, as well as from the gut to the brain.

This physiology explains why being passed over for a promotion ruins your appetite for dinner or why negative emotions result in stomach pain and discomfort, even constipation.

Stress also makes the gut (like the rest of the body) more vulnerable to infection and inflammation. These conditions can produce pain, gas, bleeding, nausea, diarrhea, and other symptoms.

The gut also manufactures important neurotransmitters, including the feel-good chemical, serotonin. Most people believe that serotonin is made in the brain, but now we know that 90 percent of it is produced in the digestive tract. Serotonin plays multiple roles in the body, influencing everything from mood to sleep to gut function. Compromised quantities of serotonin are associated with diseases, such as irritable bowel syndrome, cardiovascular disease, and osteoporosis.

Of the microorganisms populating the microbiome, the bacteria are of vital importance. They communicate through the gut to the nervous system to the brain, and its cross-talk that goes back and forth. Much of the conversation has to do with pain. Gut bacteria can adjust to how we feel pain and how well the gut works.

Decrease your stress and you will protect yourself from disease and advanced aging. The keys to managing stress and preserving health are found in the next chapter.

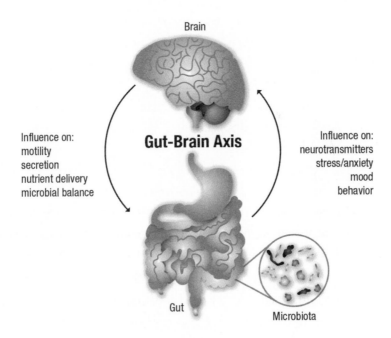

Anti-Aging Pioneer: Candace Pert, PhD

In the early 1980s, Candice Pert, PhD, concluded experiments that showed that your thoughts can have an effect on chemical changes in your body. This led to her groundbreaking book, *The Molecules of Emotion*, and the field of psychoendocrinology was born. Her work gave credence to the fact that the mind and body are not disconnected, as was believed as far back as the Middle Ages.

As this new field of medicine grew and even evolved there was more evidence that the central nervous system was also involved. The idea that a thought or an emotion can send this signal through the central nervous system's sympathetic or parasympathetic network led to an even greater discovery that it was affecting our immune cellular function. This ever-expanding field is now known as psycho-neuro-endocrine-immunology. In other words, a thought not only has a chemical component, but it is transmitted through the central nervous system to effect our defense mechanism which is our immune system. So, the thoughts of anger, fear, and doubt have different chemical reactions than the thoughts of love and accomplishment. Because of such groundbreaking research, we now have a better understanding of how the mind and stress affect the nervous system, the endocrine system, and the immune system—and create disease.

Psycho-neuro-endocrine-immunology is the science of utilizing positive mental energy, including the emotion of love, to create a sound immune system. The mind and body are not separated; they are one. In the chapter 1 of this book, you'll learn my theory of the mind-body connection known as the Apollo Factor. It is a culmination of my more than forty years of experience in discovering that disease can be reversed when we reconnect and integrate mind and body healing.

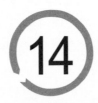

14

Solution:

AGE-DEFYING
STRESS MANAGEMENT

In the early 1990s, I treated Darrell, a fifty-year-old building contractor, for high blood pressure. While not significantly overweight and relatively young, Darrell was angry and depressed—he had recently gone through a rough divorce—and had early evidence of cardiovascular disease.

One day, my receptionist knocked on my door while I was doing hypnosis with a patient. "Darrell's here, and he doesn't look good—gray and clammy. I'm worried. I think you'd better see him now."

I have a rule in the office that if I was doing hypnotherapy with a client, to not disturb me under any circumstances. Yet, here was my receptionist knocking on the door, hard and frantically.

I hurried to the reception area. "Darrell?" I said, as he collapsed into my arms.

The receptionist called 911. I started CPR and hooked him up to an electrocardiogram. He was in a fatal type of heartbeat called ventricular fibrillation. I was in a temporary office space and had no defibrillator —a device that shocks the heart into normal rhythm. So, I resorted to the precordial thump, the medical equivalent of a Hail Mary pass in football. In other words, I thumped his chest with my fist. Hard! As I hit his chest with my fist, I yelled, "Darrell, don't you die on me! You come back now!"

A minute later, Darrell had a couple of broken ribs and a heart in normal rhythm. He opened his eyes and looked at me. "What happened?" he said. (Later, he told me that he'd been heading toward a bright light but had turned around because he had heard me yelling for him to come back.)

Darrell was awake when the EMTs arrived. To make a long story short, he'd gone into a fatal type of heart arrhythmia. At the hospital, a cardiac catheterization revealed that he needed angioplasty, a stent, or open-heart surgery to clear an artery that was nearly blocked. Back then, stents weren't placed immediately, as they are today.

While his irregular heartbeats were being stabilized in preparation for surgery, I went to the hospital to see him. I described what had happened and told him that he could try to open the artery without surgery, if he chose.

"I don't want an operation," he said. "Tell me what to do."

At his bedside, I taught him to do self-hypnosis and imagery. He spent the next thirty-six hours imagining that he was traveling with a tool he used every day in his work—a router, which makes grooves and shapes that clear the way to build new connections, and that it was clearing his blocked artery.

When the cardiac catheter was inserted a second time, in order to perform the angioplasty, Darrell's blood vessel—which had been nearly completely blocked—was now only 30 percent blocked. No surgery was needed.

What happened? I can tell you what I *think* happened. I think Darrell clotted an artery because stress and extreme anger over his divorce changed his blood chemistry. He was in a constant state of flight, in which the stress hormones, cortisol, epinephrine, and norepinephrine, were chronically elevated in his blood for months. This is called a high Beta state and signifies sympathetic nervous system overdrive. His body responded to this imbalanced chemistry by forming a clot, which in turn suddenly reduced oxygen to his heart. His electrical system created a fatal type of rhythm. His heart could not pump blood to his brain, and he almost died.

This is the same factor that Hans Selye, MD, considered by many to be the father of stress management, called the "depletion phase," precipitated by chronic depletion of the adrenals and eventually adrenal fatigue and death.

Once in the hospital, Darrell's goal was simple: "I want to live." That resolve—and the simple mind-body technique I'd taught him—sparked his psycho-immune system to be activated (the phenomenon first described by Dr. Pert). His brain was stimulated by thoughts, which in turn sent hormones to the immune system telling the body how to respond. In this case, Darrell's body dissolved a clot and reduced the injury to the heart. The clot dissolved spontaneously—a phenomenon described by Andrew Weil, MD, in his book, *Spontaneous Healing*, in the early 1990s.

I believe all disease is reversible—if you focus on the possibilities (quantum biology/physics), which means that our thoughts influence and create reality (what you believe, you conceive), rather than on the probabilities (Newtonian physics), which states that an action will probably cause a reaction. Our prevailing medical system, including the pharmaceutical industry, generally follows the Newtonian line of reasoning. A doctor listens to your symptoms, makes a diagnosis, and gives you a drug to treat it. End of story? Hardly. There is so much more to healing than this!

How to Alleviate Stress and Its Effects

The human body has many ways that it protects us from the effects of stress from our innate antioxidant response, hormone production, to our immune system, all helping us to offset the millions of impulses the nervous system has to process every day and every year. Given the controllable causes of the aging process, I believe stress management techniques provide the highest reward.

Meditation

I have often said that if I could leave a legacy to all of my patients it would be for each of them to learn the value of meditation, especially as an anti-aging strategy. People who meditate daily for five years or more add at least one productive year of life to their lives. Meditation has been found in research to reduce stress, protect the telomeres, raise telomerase, and reverse the aging process.

There are many forms of meditation and many myths regarding the practices of meditation. In some religious circles, it is believed that the meditative state is controlled by Satan or some dark force that alters the mind. Over the course of my thirty-two years of meditating, I have learned not to argue with individuals who carry a strong belief but to encourage them to find a way to induce a healing parasympathetic phase in their life.

In the Christian faith, meditation does not go against religious beliefs. Nor do I believe meditation is a form of mind control. Further, many people believe that prayer is a form of meditation, and I do not argue with them. I do, however, feel that prayer is speaking to God, while meditation is listening to the answers.

The following is a simple form of meditation that can induce all the benefits conferred by a meditative state.

- Sit in a chair that does not recline so that you do not confuse meditation with a sleep state.

- Look at a clock before you start and set your intention for ten to twenty minutes to meditate. Don't worry about the time. You can open one eye to glance briefly at the clock without interrupting your meditative state. Let no one disturb you, and turn your cell phone off.

- Close your eyes.

- Pick a mantra—a word that is meaningless to you. The mantra I choose is *samhita* (pronounced some-heat-ah). Some people like to use words like "peace," or "I am relaxed" or "I feel calm" or even a prayer like "I love the Lord."

- Say the mantra five times out loud and then keep repeating it in your head.

- Every time a thought comes into your head, say the mantra in your mind. Keep repeating the mantra if you have no thoughts.

- When the time is over, sit for at least a minute or two with your eyes closed. If you open them too suddenly, you may get a headache or a feeling of relaxation leaving your body. If that happens, close your eyes for a minute. Then slowly open them, and the headache or other odd feelings will be gone.

- Repeat this process at least ten minutes twice a day. When you awaken in the morning and at the end of your work day are the best times—but before you eat your evening meal and never as you are going to bed.

The longer you mediate, the easier it becomes and the greater its benefit—especially the feelings of rejuvenation.

A Tip from Kids

One of my mentors, George Sheehan, MD, taught me the importance of learning how to play as if I were a kid—which led me to develop what I call my "wind-up toy" technique of stress management. You know what I mean by a wind-up toy—you wind it up, it moves, and it does its thing.

I have a little alligator that opens and closes its mouth after I wind it up, and a monkey that does back flips. I have a whole collection, in fact. If some person or situation puts pressure on me—in other words is creating stress—I just imagine that person as one of my wind-up toys —and this gives me a private, stress-relieving chuckle. When I laugh, I boost natural feel-good endorphins in my system, plus I oxygenate my body. This technique works wonders, and I've used it for more than thirty-five years.

Hypnotherapy and Self-Hypnosis

While I was doing my MD and PhD studies at the University of Missouri Medical Center in Columbia, Missouri, I was part of a study group that met to advance our medical school learning experience. There, I met a young obstetrician who claimed that he could deliver babies by using a hypnotic trance rather than giving anesthesia to the mother.

He came to our group to demonstrate this method by doing group hypnosis. I said, "Are you serious? There is no way that you will be able to hypnotize me." At the time, I believed that hypnotherapy was hocus-pocus. Anyway, the demonstration began.

Fast-forward thirty minutes: I opened my eyes to the entire group, looking at me and smiling. It turned out that I did indeed fall into a trance for thirty minutes or more!

No longer skeptical, I was so impressed with the results that I later trained in hypnotherapy with Dr. Milton Erickson, a prominent American psychiatrist and psychologist who is widely regarded as the "father of hypnotherapy," and became certified as an Ericksonian hypnotherapist.

I once used hypnosis on my daughter (five years old at the time), who had chronic asthma. Afterward, she no longer had to go to the hospital with acute respiratory distress. Her asthma was better controlled with a combination of herbal medications and hypnosis than with anything else.

I then began to use hypnosis more frequently—with children in the emergency room to calm them down, in a smoking cessation program that I developed, and with my heart patients to reduce their need for pain medications after heart surgery.

You don't even have to consult a trained hypnotherapist; you can learn self-hypnosis:

- Sit in a comfortable chair in an upright position (no recliners).
- Look upward as if there is a penny on the top of your head. When you feel comfortable, close your eyelids.
- Imagine that you are going to relieve all the tension in the muscles of your neck, shoulders, upper back, arms, and face. Let all that tension release down through your forearms and out of your body through your fingertips, as you slowly count down from 10–9–8–7–6–5–4–3–2–1.
- Repeat this sequence with other muscles in your lower back, hips, buttocks, thighs, hamstrings, and calves. Allow the tension in these muscles to travel down your legs and out the body through your toes as you slowly count down from 10–9–8–7–6–5–4–3–2–1.
- With your eyes still closed, go to a safe, calm place in your mind—a nice room in your house, your backyard, the beach, or the mountains, and so forth. Imagine that you are actually

there, noticing objects you have not seen before. Let you mind relax as you look around; give the image a name. Slowly count down from 10–9–8–7–6–5–4–3–2–1 as you feel more relaxed with fewer intrusive thoughts and no muscle tension. Stay in this state for a minute or more.

- Now begin to slowly count from 1 to 5 as you become more aware of your present surroundings. You will find that you are alert, but it will be difficult to open your eyes. Don't try to force it; eventually, they will open. You'll "awake," feeling energized and refreshed.

It also helps to do this exercise by listening to a voice recording and following the instructions.

Yoga and Tai Chi

I covered these in chapter 10, but I want to emphasize them here, too. Both are "moving meditations," known to help lower your stress hormones and put your body and mind back into synchronicity. Yoga, in particular, increases telomere length, especially if you can stay in the pose known as corpse pose, in which you lie on your back, eyes closed, arms at your sides, and palms pointed upward.

I always suggest yoga as a way to increase relaxation, help with anti-aging, and stimulate a parasympathetic experience. Gentle, non-aggressive forms of yoga are best.

The true, underlying goal of tai chi is to harness the *qi*, or life energy, within us so that it can flow smoothly and powerfully throughout the body. The best way to practice the movements of tai chi, in my opinion, is to hold the poses and move slowly. Combining certain breathing techniques and holding certain meditative poses induces a type of meditation. (See chapter 16 on the Apollo Factor for more ways to cultivate your life energy.)

Tai chi is probably one of the best modes of exercise for anyone who suffers from major imbalances, especially after neurologic compromise and strokes. Tai chi classes have sprung up throughout the United States, even in hospitals.

Look to Ayurveda for Stress Relief

Practitioners of Ayurveda follow a daily routine that eases stress, and I have modeled my 7-day plan after this. Their routine includes:

- Waking up early (usually at the same time before the sun rises);
- Meditating prior to work, and a second time later in the day;
- Performing gentle exercise, such as yoga;
- Nurturing the body with a light meal;
- Going to work;
- Taking midday break;
- Sitting quietly to enjoy lunch and later, dinner;
- Relaxing after work;
- Retiring to bed early.

The reason this routine helps alleviate stress is because the body runs on a clock of sorts, the so-called circadian rhythm, in which our physiological processes are synced to the twenty-four-hour solar cycle of light and dark. Since prehistoric times, the circadian rhythm has regulated the pattern of being awake by day and sleeping by night. It does this by governing the timing of the brain's release of cortisol and other hormones. The part of the brain governing your circadian rhythm is the *suprachiasmatic nucleus*, a clump of nerves at the center of the brain—and it loves predictability.

A regular schedule or routine is thus essential to help *you* manage daily stress. If you approach your day with some sort of plan of action, you'll experience less stress.

NuCalm

In my practice, I use a clinical system called NuCalm to help the mind and body relax naturally in minutes. It is especially effective as a way to treat patients with post-traumatic stress disorder, brought on by accidents, abuse, combat, and other traumatic life events—and one of the best ways to achieve the parasympathetic state.

With this system, you sit comfortably in a dark room. A special calming cream is applied to your temples, and an FDA-approved cranial electrotherapy device is attached to your head. You also put on a light-blocking eye mask to eliminate any visual stimuli and help you reach a state of deep relaxation. Special frequencies are delivered to your brain, which bring on theta brain waves, a state of deep relaxation. Theta brain waves increase heart rate variability (HRV), the beat-to-beat fluctuations in heart rate. When you are feeling calm and relaxed, HRV is elevated, and you can more effortlessly manage stress. In healthy people, HRV is high. A high HRV determines your cardiovascular health, your fitness level, and even your longevity.

The entire session takes only twenty to thirty minutes. Afterward, you feel rested and focused—a result of your cells being cleansed and restored. To find a NuCalm provider in your area, check out *www.nucalm.com.*

Healing Sound

In the mid-1970s, I became interested in the use of sound frequencies to treat disease, after reading studies showing that certain types of music could change the way a plant grew. I wondered that if music could affect plant growth, why couldn't it influence cellular function and possibly bring about healing?

I theorized that we are born in perfect vibration and that toxic environmental influences put us out of tune. When the cells vibrate to the wrong frequency, mitochondrial dysfunction occurs, affecting our organs and thus allowing disease to grab a foothold. If we could restore our cosmic tune, disease might disappear. I called this "the theory of our cosmic song."

Then I met a soon-to-be friend named Michael Tyrrell, who had conducted fascinating research on vibrational sounds in healing. Michael is a brilliant and accomplished musician, composer, inventor, and producer. He explained to me that everything possesses a resonant frequency (which reminded me of our cosmic tune). Resonance occurs when a physical system is periodically disturbed at the same period as one of its natural frequencies—but that by listening to certain frequencies, a person can begin to heal from PTSD, depression, anxiety, hearing loss, or just to feel more calm. Michael went on to create Wholetones, a musical series on CDs, designed to bring you into the relaxing parasympathetic state. For those again who will or cannot experience a meditative state, feel free to investigate vibration as a healing technology at *www.whole tones.com*.

Music therapy is used as a complementary treatment for dementia, psychological stress, anxiety, substance abuse, stroke, and pain, among other conditions. You can harness the power of music in your own life to reduce stress; as long as you listen to calming music and not heavy-metal music (research shows it abnormally reduces heart rate variability!). You'll discover that the right music can quickly ease tension and put you in a more positive mood that in turn helps you cope better with stressors. So, let music into your life!

Quantum Physics, Thoughts, and Active Imagery

Quantum thought, based on quantum physics, simply means that what you think becomes reality. In the case of my patients Darrell (earlier in this chapter) and Phil (chapter 4), they used a quantum thought called "active imagery—a router cleaning out a clot from his artery. Basically, this involved the conscious directed use of the imagination to activate a healing response. Other examples might be Pac-men gobbling up tumors or imagining you as a warrior defeating a disease. Research has confirmed that this practice boosts the production and proper functioning of immune cells, including T cells and natural killer cells. I believe that active imagery is powerful and should be an adjunct therapy in all cases of illness and disease.

Quantum thought definitely helps avert stress. Your thoughts can unleash a flood of stress hormones. When you experience scary or anxious thoughts, for example, your brain reacts and tells the adrenal glands to pump out stress hormones—even though the scary or anxious thought is only in your head. The brain can't differentiate whether threats are real or imagined. In either case, the physical consequences are the same: adrenaline is released, you feel anxious, your heart rate increases, your palms sweat, and breathing picks up.

Suppose you're about to go into a high-pressure situation, say a job interview. If you tell yourself internally, "I'm going to blow it; I'll be terrible," your brain will believe it, because what the conscious mind states, the unconscious mind will provide via hormones.

With these thoughts come the stammering, trembling, or emotional paralysis once you get in the interview. Those toxic thoughts acted as a stress to the body that then unbalances your stress hormones, making you feel anxious, shy, and easily intimidated. Your prophetic thoughts manifest, and you do, indeed, blow the interview. In a case like this, what you think has truly altered your reality.

But just as our thoughts can trigger a stress response, they can also create calm, healing experiences, too. For example, if you imagine yourself performing well in the interview, it's as if the brain says to the body, "It's okay; you can relax now." Positive thoughts release endorphins that make you feel good and reduce stress hormones—and this may result in your being hired for that job, or at least you'll feel better about your interview performance.

It's healthier and more productive to be optimistic, especially when you are facing adversity. Many studies have demonstrated that a generally positive attitude is much healthier than a pessimistic one, and that optimists not only feel better mentally, but are even more likely to resist disease and heal faster. (For more information on this, see chapter 16 regarding the Apollo Factor.)

Applying positive quantum thought could fill up several books, but let me provide some suggestions:

- Instead of tearing yourself down, build yourself up when things aren't going as expected. Turn negatives into positives: You're not unemployed, you're just between jobs. You're not broke, you financially challenged and on your way back.
- Don't ask, "Why me?" Substitute "why" for "how." "How can I make it better? How can I improve my finances? How can I get in shape?" Ask these questions, and then answer them.
- Past-tense unproductive thoughts. Telling yourself "I'll never lose weight" or "I'll never get a promotion" only makes these doubts more of a reality. Reframe this kind of self-talk and think of your perceived shortcomings as if they had happened in the past, rather than the present or future. For example: "I've never been able to lose weight" or "I used to be in a lower-ranking job." This technique helps you feel more positive about your life and future.
- Dispute automatic negative thoughts. Every moment of every day, "automatic thoughts" flit through your mind. They tend to be self-evaluations, such as "I can't do this" or "I can do this." These thoughts trigger the release stress hormones and elicit emotional reactions that cause distress.

  Whenever you feel sad, mad, or nervous, you need to write out what you are thinking, and look at it analytically. Ask yourself:

"Is this true, or am I just torturing myself unnecessarily?" You don't have to believe every thought you have. Thoughts can lie. Correct them or replace them with truer, more positive thoughts, and the stress induced by negative thinking will switch off.

- Consume your mind with so many positives that you don't have time to think about the negatives. Positive thoughts lead to positive feelings that allow us to filter in all good things.

Laugh Often and Much

Norman Cousins, an editor at the *Saturday Review*, was struck with ankylosing spondylitis, a degenerative disease of the connective tissue, after a stressful trip to Russia. Reasoning that laughter could have a healing effect, he watched hours of Marx Brothers movies, the Three Stooges, and Abbott and Costello clips. One of the things Cousins discovered was that a ten-minute belly laugh helped him sleep without pain. Many other studies have shown that feel-good endorphins are released as a result of laughter, and they may ease the pain in those suffering from arthritis, spondylitis, and muscular spasms.

Then why aren't doctors shouting the "laughter cure" from the rooftops? Answer: They are too busy trying to make a living and seeing fifty to sixty patients a day. They don't laugh themselves! Why would they teach you a technique they do not know how to use in their own lives?

Bottom line: Laugh more and live longer.

These stress management techniques can control our nutritional habits, as well as the use or abuse of substances like alcohol and drugs, both prescription and recreational. What's more, they lower the hormones that cause oxidation and inflammation and repair the body's protective immune system. The happier and more stress-free you are, the longer you will live.

(15)

THE 7-DAY
REJUVENATION PLAN

You can start living a healthier, more youthful life today. I've developed a 7-Day Rejuvenation Plan to jump-start your anti-aging lifestyle. It helps you take just a few simple anti-aging steps every day to put you on the path of a healthier future and cut your risk of age-related illnesses.

Although the plan covers just seven days, don't limit yourself to trying it for a week. These daily guidelines are healthy, age-reversing habits that you can keep up for life.

Once you've completed these seven days, repeat for another week, and another, adapting the plan for your lifestyle. It puts all of my seven anti-aging solutions into action and is the perfect plan for the rest of your life.

Let's get started.

Prepping for the Plan

1. Go to the grocery store and stock up on a week's worth of anti-aging foods. Some suggestions:

Vegetables: Green leafy veggies such as kale, spinach, spring greens, and lettuce; broccoli, cauliflower, and Brussels sprouts; green beans; salad vegetables (onions, tomatoes, sprouts, cucumbers, and so forth; bell peppers; summer squash and zucchini; and any of your favorite vegetables. The more colorful the vegetables, the better.

Fruit: berries of all types, citrus fruits, peaches, pears, plums, and cantaloupe.

Fresh herbs: rosemary, basil, sage, parsley, thyme, and so forth.

Vegetable proteins: beans, legumes, lentils, almond milk yogurt, and nut milks.

Whole grains: oatmeal, quinoa, brown rice, and barley.

Nuts and seeds: almonds, cashews, Brazil nuts, pecans, walnuts, chia seeds, flaxseeds, sunflower seeds, pumpkin seeds, and so forth.

Oils: olive oil, coconut oil.

Olives: organic, pitted black and green olives.

2. See an integrative physician (MD, DO, DC, ND, or TCM) about having specific laboratory tests related to anti-aging. You can locate physicians in your area on the website acam.org. Lab tests to consider are:

Complete Blood Count (CBC)

Fasting Glucose Test

HgA1C

Fasting Insulin

Oxidation (SpectraCell) or Cleveland heart labs

C-Reactive Protein

Vitamin C

B12

Serum Folate

Hormone Panel

Telomere testing (Life Length)

Based on the results of your testing, the physician may prescribe bioidentical hormones and make recommendations for specific nutritional supplements to take.

3. Head to your favorite health food store or pharmacy and stock up on my recommended supplements. You don't have to take every single one; choices depend on the current state of your health. Everyone, however, should follow the Basic Anti-Aging Supplement Plan. If you have specific conditions such as diabetes, heart disease, joint problems, or others, follow the Therapeutic Supplement Plan, in addition to the Basic Supplement Plan. Here are the guidelines:

Basic Anti-Aging Supplement Plan

Antioxidant multiple vitamin and mineral supplement: Take one supplement daily.

Vitamin C: 1250–5000 milligrams daily

Alpha lipoic acid: 600 to 1200 milligrams daily

Astaxanthin: 4 to 12 milligrams daily

CoQ10: 200 to 400 milligrams daily. If you're taking statins, or have known heart disease, high blood pressure, or cancer, take 400 to 800 milligrams daily

Green tea extract: Two to three cups daily of brewed green tea; or 150 to 2500 milligrams of green tea extract in divided dosages

Quercetin: 100 to 250 milligrams three times a day

Resveratrol: 250 to 1000 milligrams daily

Clary sage oil (for omega-3 fatty acids): 2 tablespoons daily

Probiotic supplement: 1 or 2 capsules daily (50 billion colonies)

Zinc: 15–30 milligrams daily

B complex supreme: one capsule daily (follow manufacturer's recommendation for dosage

Carnosine: 500 milligrams daily

Vitamin D3: 2000–10000 IU's daily

Magnesium: 200 to 400 milligrams of magnesium daily, preferably at night, because this mineral helps with sleep

Therapeutic Supplement Plan

This plan is designed to support the treatment of specific conditions, many of which are age-related—diabetes, liver damage, coronary artery disease, joint problems, and so forth. Take the following supplements in addition to the supplements listed above, and according to your individual health needs.

Alpha lipoic acid: increase dosage if you have diabetes, liver damage, or coronary artery disease to 1500 to 2000 milligrams daily.

Glutathione (diabetes, liver damage, coronary artery disease, lung problems, Parkinson's disease): glutathione drips of 2000 to 4000 milligrams given in drips several times monthly.

L-citrulline (muscle loss in elderly, heart disease): 3 to 6 grams taken with 1500 milligrams to 3 grams of arginine.

Turmeric extract: for osteoarthritis: 500 milligrams twice daily for two to three months; for high cholesterol: 700 milligrams twice daily for three months; for itchy skin: 500 milligrams three times daily for two months.

Aged garlic extract: for hardening of the arteries: 250 milligrams taken daily; for diabetes: 600 to 1500 milligrams daily; for high cholesterol: 1000 to 7200 milligrams daily in divided doses; for high blood pressure: 960 to 7200 milligrams, taken daily in up to three divided doses

DHEA: 50 to 100 milligrams orally in the morning if hormone testing indicates you need it. For women suffering from chronic fatigue or cortisol imbalances, I might up that dosage to 100 to 300 milligrams of DHEA.

TA-65: If telomere testing reveals that you have shortened telomeres, take two to six capsules daily. If your test reveals the highest number of short telomeres, for example, you'd supplement at the higher range.

4. Look up the closest yoga, Pilates, or tai chi center. Call and sign up for the first class that fits your schedule.

ANTI-AGING PLAN: Day 1

---

6 AM: Wake up. There's no universal wake-up time that fits everyone, but it's ideal to rise when your body is best prepared—at the conclusion of our deepest sleep, called rapid eye movement (REM) sleep, which occurs before we naturally wake up. Usually, this will happen after about seven to eight hours of sleep.

7–8 AM: Eat within one to two hours of waking. Start your day with a bowl of cooked oatmeal, one-half cup of almond milk—topped with sliced strawberries and two tablespoons of chopped almonds, along with a cup of green or herbal tea.

After breakfast, get some sunlight if possible. The best time to go outdoors is within two hours of waking up. The UV component of sunlight is low, but the bright light sets you on a good course of alertness.

9 AM: Organize your workflow for the day to avoid feeling stressed out and overwhelmed. Once you've laid out your to-do list, get to work. Make this a daily morning habit.

10 AM: Spend ten to twenty minutes in meditation. Follow this with a mid-morning snack, such as a piece of fruit.

12–1 PM: Have a large salad with lots of raw vegetables, including leafy greens, tossed in an olive oil–based dressing.

Late afternoon or after work: Attend a yoga, Pilates, or tai chi class. (Many people like to work out in the morning. If you're one of them, feel free to do so.

For an afternoon snack, have a piece of fruit with a few nuts or seeds.

6–7 PM: Enjoy a meatless dinner tonight: at least six ounces of a vegetable protein with two cooked vegetables of different colors. Have a small tossed salad, too.

Throughout the day: Take your daily supplements as recommended—and hormones if prescribed.

Hydrate: Drink at least eight glasses of alkaline water throughout the day. When you're hydrated, you'll feel more energized, be less likely to give into cravings, and stimulate a more functional metabolism.

10 PM: Bedtime. Starting on Day 1, set a consistent bedtime rather than varying your routine every night. A predictable bedtime prepares your body and mind for restorative sleep and helps to regulate your body's clock for hormone balance.

ANTI-AGING PLAN: Day 2

6 AM: Wake up.

7–8 AM: Make a fruit smoothie for breakfast with one cup blueberries, one-half cup strawberries, one-half banana, and a handful of spinach.

If possible, get some daylight right after breakfast.

9 AM: Organize your workflow for the day.

10 AM: Spend ten to twenty minutes in meditation. Follow this with a mid-morning snack, such as a piece of fruit.

12–1 PM: Have a large salad with lots of raw vegetables for lunch, tossed in an olive oil–based dressing.

Late afternoon or after work: Go for a walk in nature for twenty to thirty minutes. Research confirms that spending just twenty minutes outside in good weather not only improves mood, but it sharpens thinking and memory. If the weather is bad, find an indoor mall or walk the halls (and stairs) of your office building if it's large enough.

For an afternoon snack, have a piece of fruit or raw veggies dipped in hummus.

6–7 PM: Enjoy another meatless dinner tonight: Sauté veggies, such as onions, slices of orange, red, and green bell peppers, and mushrooms, and serve them over cooked brown rice or riced cauliflower—along with a side salad. Dinners like these add a layer of protection against contributors to aging: oxidative stress, chronic inflammation, shortened telomeres, and unbalanced hormones.

Throughout the day: Take your daily supplements as recommended—and hormones if prescribed.

Hydrate: Drink at least eight glasses of alkaline water throughout the day.

10 PM: Bedtime. Start new bedtime habits for quality sleep. For example, take electronics (including your TV) out of the room. Listen to some soft music or read a book, rather than watching TV. Either will be easier on your eyes than a television or tablet.

ANTI-AGING PLAN: Day 3

---

6 AM: Wake up.

7–8 AM: Try intermittent fasting today in which you do not eat anything between last night's dinner and this morning. (Go for fourteen to sixteen hours without eating.) Rather than your usual breakfast, have a cup of hot water with lemon juice or a cup of herbal tea. Intermittent fasting helps you restrict calories—a proven anti-aging strategy.

If possible, get some daylight right after breakfast.

9 AM: Organize your workflow for the day.

10 AM: Spend ten to twenty minutes in meditation. Follow this with a snack, such as a piece of fruit and a cup of almond milk yogurt.

12–1 PM: Fix veggie wraps with two large lettuce leaves. Spread with mashed avocado and fill with sprouts, tomato slices, and cucumber slices.

At work, try to get up from your desk and move around. Every two hours of sitting increases the risk of type 2 diabetes by 7 percent and heart disease by 25 percent. Moving more and sitting less will keep your bones strong.

Late afternoon or after work: Do full-body strength training routine for thirty to forty-five minutes. For an afternoon snack, have a handful of nuts and a piece of fruit.

6–7 PM: Chop a couple of Portobello mushrooms and cook them in marina sauce. Serve over cooked spaghetti squash, along with a tossed salad.

Throughout the day: Take your daily supplements as recommended—and hormones if prescribed.

Hydrate: Drink at least eight glasses of alkaline water throughout the day.

10 PM: Bedtime. Turn off the television and computer, put the pile of work away, and take a warm bath prior to going to bed. Remember to keep electronics out of your bedroom for better sleep quality. The blue light from tablets, laptops, and smart phones interferes with falling asleep because it suppresses melatonin, an essential hormone for sleep.

ANTI-AGING PLAN: Day 4

6 AM: Wake up.

7–8 AM: Continue intermittent fasting today. (Go for fourteen to sixteen hours without eating.) Rather than your usual breakfast, have a cup of hot water with lemon juice or a cup of herbal tea.

If possible, get some daylight right after breakfast.

9 AM: Organize your workflow for the day.

10 AM: Spend ten to twenty minutes in meditation. Follow this with a mid-morning snack, such as a handful of nuts and a piece of fruit.

12–1 PM: Have a large bowl of bean or lentil soup with a tossed side salad.

Late afternoon or after work: Attend a yoga, Pilates, or tai chi class. For an afternoon snack, have a piece of fruit. For an afternoon snack, have a fruit smoothie.

6–7 PM: Enjoy a huge dinner salad with spinach and kale as the base, topped with vegan cheese, sunflower seeds, chickpeas, chopped avocado, and cherry tomatoes, tossed with an olive oil-based dressing.

Throughout the day: Take your daily supplements as recommended—and hormones if prescribed.

Hydrate: Drink at least eight glasses of alkaline water throughout the day.

10 PM: Bedtime. If you're having trouble getting to sleep, drink a cup of sleepy-time herbal tea or 1 cup of almond milk warmed with one-half teaspoon ghee and cinnamon.

ANTI-AGING PLAN: Day 5

6 AM: Wake up.

7–8 AM: Continue intermittent fasting today. (Go for fourteen to sixteen hours without eating.) Rather than your usual breakfast, have a cup of hot water with lemon juice or a cup of herbal tea.

If possible, get some daylight right after breakfast.

9 AM: Organize your workflow for the day.

10 AM: Spend ten to twenty minutes in meditation. Follow this with a mid-morning snack, such as a bowl of cut-up fruit and a handful of walnuts (antioxidants, fiber, protein, and healthy fats all rolled up into one).

12–1 PM: Have a large salad with lots of raw vegetables for lunch, tossed in an olive oil–based dressing.

Start a new habit at lunch: Use your lunchtime (no matter how limited it may be) to refuel not only your body but also your mind: Read or listen to some inspirational materials.

Late afternoon or after work: Go for a walk in nature for twenty to thirty minutes. If the weather is bad, find an indoor mall or walk the halls (and stairs) of your office building if it's large enough. For an afternoon snack, have a piece of fruit or raw veggies dipped in hummus.

6–7 PM: Enjoy some cauliflower/veggie pizza slices with a tossed salad.

Throughout the day: Take your daily supplements as recommended—and hormones if prescribed.

Hydrate: Drink at least eight glasses of alkaline water throughout the day.

10 PM: Bedtime. Make your bedroom be cool—between sixty-five and sixty-eight degrees—and free from noise and light.

ANTI-AGING PLAN: Day 6

6 AM: Wake up.

7–8 AM: Have a cup of almond milk yogurt with live cultures with a tablespoon of ground flaxseeds sprinkled on top, along with a piece of fruit. The probiotics in the yogurt enhance your immune system and reduce toxin absorption. The flaxseeds provide blood sugar–reducing fiber and omega-3 fatty acids that fight inflammation.

If possible, get some daylight right after breakfast.

10 AM: Spend ten to twenty minutes in meditation. Follow this with a mid-morning snack, such as a piece of fruit.

12–1 PM: Have a black bean burger with tossed salad and a piece of fresh fruit.

Late afternoon or after work: Do full-body strength training routine for thirty to forty-five minutes. For an afternoon snack, have a piece of fruit or raw veggies dipped in hummus.

6–7 PM: Enjoy a plant-based meal out at a restaurant. Then go out with a friend or loved one and watch a comedy at the movie theater.

Throughout the day: Take your daily supplements as recommended—and hormones if prescribed.

Hydrate: Drink at least eight glasses of alkaline water throughout the day.

10 PM: Bedtime. Prior to going to sleep, make a list of what you're grateful for. This is one of the simplest ways to relieve stress, fight depression, and foster happiness—and much research supports what I'm recommending. This "gratitude habit" is a good one to do most nights of the week.

ANTI-AGING PLAN: Day 7

6 AM: Wake up.

7–8 AM: Make a fruit smoothie for breakfast with one cup blueberries, one-half cup strawberries, one-half banana, and one handful of spinach.

If possible, get some daylight right after breakfast. Spend ten to twenty minutes in meditation. Follow this with a mid-morning snack, such as a piece of fruit.

12–1 PM: Have a large salad with lots of raw vegetables for lunch, tossed in an olive oil–based dressing.

Late afternoon or after work: Go for a walk in nature for twenty to thirty minutes. If the weather is bad, find an indoor mall.

For an afternoon snack, have a piece of fruit or raw veggies dipped in hummus.

6–7 PM: Sauté a mix of different types of mushrooms—Portobello, shiitake, and chanterelle with minced garlic in olive oil. Serve over butternut squash fettuccine, and have a tossed side salad.

Throughout the day: Take your daily supplements as recommended—and hormones if prescribed.

Hydrate: Drink at least eight glasses of alkaline water throughout the day.

10 PM: Bedtime. Tip: Don't drink alcohol at night; it may make you sleepy, but it interferes with quality, restorative sleep.

Please feel free to modify the schedule to accomplish your goals. I often change the schedule around on weekends by starting with meditation and then having a plant-based protein shake and going for a motorcycle ride before I go to the gym. Even though the schedule looks a little rigid, use your imagination to be successful, play, and have fun on your quest to slow down the causes of aging.

16

THE APOLLO FACTOR: RECLAIM YOUR COSMIC GIFT OF SELF-HEALING

Within each of us is the potential of the body to self-heal and increase our life span and health span. This potential is the force behind spontaneous healing—the disappearance of symptoms without formal treatment—the infinite wisdom of the body and its vast armies to conquer illness and extend life, and the wondrous power of the mind-body connection to make us well.

I call this force, or system, the Apollo Factor, named after the Greek god, Apollo, who among other responsibilities was the god of healing.

The Apollo Factor encompasses every solution to aging and disease that I have talked about in this book, including plant-based nutrition and medicinal herbs, Ayurveda and other ancient medical practices, meditation and relaxation, physical exercise, quantum physics and thought, and epigenetics—along with my decades of experience as both physician and healer (basically nothing we doctors learn in medical school!).

When you ignite the Apollo Factor with positive, conscious messages from the mind, it improves health and helps prevent disease at the cellular level. In this final section of the book, I will explore with you how to do this, bringing together the seven solutions for self-healing and longevity. Learning to use the Apollo Factor can return you to a state of perfect health.

How the Apollo Factor Works: A Bridge to Healing

We have two bodies—one made of flesh, blood, and bone, and the other of energy. The Apollo Factor connects these two bodies, much like a bridge connects two spans of land. When that connection is strong, health is optimal. When that connection is weak, illness can take hold.

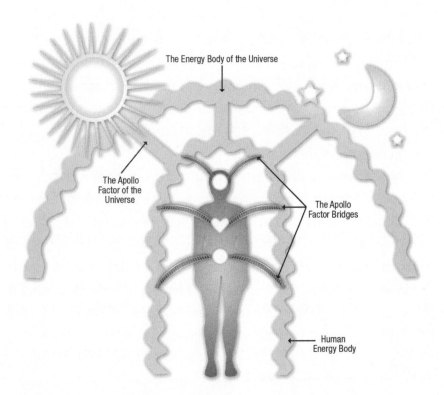

Imagine for a moment one of two famous American bridges—the Golden Gate in San Francisco or the Verrazano-Narrows in New York—both of which you've likely seen in photos or crossed in your travels.

On postcards, these suspension bridges sweep gracefully across a night sky, glittering with lights. What you can't see from the postcards is that these light, flexible bridges have roadways that literally hang from strong, yet flexible steel cables.

I've run across the Verrazano during the New York City Marathon and ridden my Harley across the Golden Gate. And let me tell you, these bridges *move*, both up and down and sideways. You can actually feel them sway and vibrate—energy in constant, gentle motion. That's the Apollo Factor—the bridge that connects mind and body, made not of steel, but pure energy.

The Apollo Factor and Healing

Take any ailment you can think of: depression, migraines, high blood pressure, obesity, or digestive issues. I've treated people with all of them, and they've recovered. Actually, all I did was teach them techniques and remedies that they then used to signal the body to heal.

How does the Apollo Factor affect body-wide healing? I propose that when stimulated by positive, conscious messages from the mind, the Apollo Factor promotes health and helps prevent the onset of disease at the cellular level.

Far-fetched? Not for a shaman. I've been exploring the Apollo Factor since my early days as a surgeon. Over and over, I saw things that I just couldn't understand, even with my training and experience. People, who should have recovered, died. People, who were definitely terminally ill, got well. There didn't appear to be logical explanations. Were they miracles? The physician and researcher in me began to look for mechanisms or an explanation for this phenomenon.

Take spontaneous healing (or as the medical literature now calls it, "spontaneous regression"), for example. How does it occur? Theories are plentiful; proof, not so much. A recent study by the famed Mayo Clinic named this phenomenon spontaneous regression. Possible explanations for spontaneous regression include increased apoptosis and necrosis (forms of cell death), epigenetic modifications, hormonal responses, cytokines, and psychological mechanisms.

In other words, no one knows what triggers spontaneous healing. And while it's real, the term implies that there's no order to the process, but I don't believe that's true. The one thing I and Western doctors can agree on is that it isn't caused by a miracle, but by a mechanism. The Apollo Factor is that mechanism.

The Apollo Factor and
Your Energy Body

In the 1970s, I observed how different types of music (vibrations) caused plants to either thrive or wither. I failed to realize what is obvious to me now: the healing system of a living thing *does not reside in its physical body*, but that was the only place I looked.

To understand what I mean, try this little experiment: Close your eyes. Turn your palm away from your face, and then hold it right in front of your nose, with fingers spread. Slowly, push your hand away from your face. At some point, your fingers will tingle, and you'll feel resistance. That's your energy body you sense. It's central to healing, and remember that the Apollo Factor is the energetic bridge that tethers it to the physical body. Heal your energy body, and your physical body will follow.

Allusions to the energy body are found in the traditions of indigenous healers worldwide—the Aborigines in Australia, the tribal peoples of India, the Native Americans of North America, and the Q'ero Shaman of Peru. It plays a central role in the processes of health and disease, and is affected even before symptoms or disease manifest. Properly activated, the Apollo Factor retunes our DNA to its unique "song," and restores us to perfect or near perfect health. And the energy body helps explain the origin of what I call our "cosmic song."

Your Cosmic Song

Each of us has a unique vibration—a "song" bestowed by the universe at the moment of our conception. That song is in our DNA—the molecule that holds the universal code of life, the genetic blueprint encoded in our trillions of cells that determines our physical characteristics, propensity for disease, and, to a certain extent, metabolic processes.

The Apollo Factor is your song's "conductor." As it transmits your DNA's vibration to your cells, the energy body retunes your DNA and can change your life at the physical level by directly resetting your DNA to vibrate to your song. Your body can begin to sing it again, returning to perfect harmony.

We enter the world in perfect health, our bodies singing their singular songs in perfect pitch. After birth, however, our cells and organs sustain damage from the two environments in which we live. The first environment, our internal "landscape," encompasses our thoughts, emotions, beliefs, and memories. The second, our external surroundings, include the food we eat, toxic chemicals in the air and water, and overexposure to electromagnetic fields.

Bad food and bad relationships, polluted air and simmering anger, chemical-laden water and too much stress, electromagnetic signals from cell phones, computers, tablets, and TV—all can cause our cells and organs to sing out of tune. If we're only a bit out of tune, we might get a cold, an injury, a pain, or some other warning sign not yet a true symptom of disease. If seriously out of tune, we may develop more severe symptoms or diseases. Serious genetic disharmony can manifest in the body as chronic inflammation.

In an ideal world, your DNA would stay in rhythm with that song, in harmony with your energy body. Because your Apollo Factor is fully activated, your energy and physical bodies would be in tune, and your health would improve.

To make that happen, one of the things we do is repair what I call *wormholes*—areas of damage in the energy body inflicted by our internal and external environments. Left untreated, wormholes can lead to imbalances of the physical body and eventually to disease. Strengthening the Apollo Factor with the simple and natural techniques in this book helps repair health-damaging wormholes, thereby returning the physical body to optimum health.

I have seen this happen time and time again—when the Apollo Factor is strengthened in my patients. They have improved and even reversed type 2 diabetes, cancer, and heart disease. And all I do is help my patients "remember" and activate their Apollo Factor with all of the strategies you have learned here.

The Apollo Factor and the Mind

Think of your mind as an iceberg in the ocean. The small part visible above the waves is the *conscious* mind, which we use every day to perceive, think, feel, and act—to carry on the business of life. The bulk of the iceberg, unseen beneath the waves, is the *unconscious* mind—the storehouse of memory, the source of intuition and dreams, the engine that powers much of the brain's information processing.

The power of the unconscious mind lies in its enormous and untapped energy. That's that nonphysical energy harnessed by the sages of the past and used to heal. Our unconscious minds exert a powerful influence on our thoughts, emotions, and behaviors, which studies show affect our physical health.

The Apollo Factor engages both the conscious and unconscious minds, an alliance that makes the mind even more powerful. If you want to lose weight or kick smoking—or beat cancer, for that matter—you want to do it with awareness and intent. Because it's your conscious level of awareness that augments the stored energy of your unconscious.

You see the Apollo Factor at work in the research conducted by Dean Ornish, MD, whose intensive cardiac rehabilitation program has been shown to actually reverse heart disease. His research, now replicated by other researchers in the field of epigenetics, shows that lifestyle changes—including meditation and yoga—can affect gene expression. That is, they "turn on" disease-preventing genes and "turn off" genes that promote cancer and heart disease. The cardiac rehabilitation program I headed in the 1980s took a similar approach, using nutrition, exercise, and stress management through meditative practice and visualization to both heal their hearts and show them a healthier way to live.

To activate the Apollo Factor, heal the energy body, and affect physical healing, the mind must be fully open and aware. The Buddha said, "We are formed and molded by our thoughts." That was more than 2000 years ago, and modern science is just now starting to prove him right. The late neuroscientist Candace Pert, PhD, wrote that "the molecules of our emotions share intimate connections with, and are indeed inseparable from, our physiology... consciously, or more frequently, unconsciously, we choose how we feel at every single moment." These "intimate connections" describe the Apollo Factor. Implicit in her words is the idea that our thoughts determine our physiology—that the mind affects outcomes of health and disease.

Techniques that balance the mind and emotions repair wormholes in the energy body and ignite the Apollo Factor. Indeed, research conducted by Herbert Benson, MD, founder of the Mind/Body Medical Institute at Massachusetts General Hospital, and Larry Dossey, MD, author of *Prayer Is Good Medicine*, has validated the efficacy of meditation, prayer, and breathing exercises—practices once prescribed by priests, shamans, and yogis—to treat chronic diseases from type 2 diabetes and heart disease to autoimmune diseases like irritable bowel syndrome.

If the Apollo Factor isn't working at full capacity, physical health is at risk. Repeated adverse events—whether emotional or physical wounds—can disrupt the healing process or thwart it altogether. My program focuses on strengthening the Apollo Factor so that it can correct the wormholes, thereby returning the physical body to perfect balance and health. Put another way, on my plan, you learn to teach your mind to work with body to effect healing.

Perhaps you're ready to believe in the mind's potent ability to heal, but you have one more question. That question: What's the *source* of mind's power?

Energy.

Harness the Healing Energy of the Universe

Many non-Western healing systems assume the existence of an energy in every living thing—people, animals, plants. Shamans call this "life force" *kawsi;* the Japanese, *ki;* and the Chinese call it *qi.* In Ayurvedic medicine, *prana* permeates the body, and you can ingest it in much the same way as a nutrient in food. Interestingly, this idea is similar to the one I had in the 1970s, when it struck me that food is energy. That epiphany led me to focus more on the energy of healing, rather than the physical body.

In traditional Chinese medicine, this vital energy, called *qi* (pronounced "chi") flows through energy pathways (*meridians*) in the body. Achieving the proper flow of *qi* promotes balance of body, mind, and spirit, which leads to health and well-being.

Here are some examples of the life force in action all around us:

- Plants respond to subtle vibrations of their leaves caused by the munching of insects—and raise their chemical defenses in response to this danger.
- Bees buzz at just the right frequency to release pollen from flowering plants.
- Corn roots grow toward an auditory source playing continuous tones and responded better to certain frequencies.

My thinking posits that every living thing possesses an Apollo Factor —plants, animals, humans, the universe. The idea that energies play a role in healing is as old as civilization itself, and modern studies support it.

- Prayer—which researchers call "distant healing"—posits a non-local effect: the minds of some people influence others' physical health. Research has associated group prayer with significant treatment gains in numerous disorders, including heart disease, Parkinson's disease, and even cancer, among other conditions.
- Hypnosis results in significant reductions in pain associated with a variety of chronic-pain problems, including arthritis, back pain, fibromyalgia, and cancer, an analysis of thirteen studies found.
- Meditation may reduce blood pressure. Even a scientific statement from the American Heart Association says so. It suggests that evidence supports the use of TM (Transcendental Meditation) as a complementary therapy along with standard treatment.

While the ancient healers understood the link between mind and body, and nonphysical energy played a central role in their healing philosophies and methods, they didn't have the whole picture. My Apollo Factor concurs with their concepts but also expands them.

Although they are connected, "life force" is different from the energy of the universe. The former is the body's internal energy; it dwells in the physical body. The energy of the universe exists outside of the physical body. They, too, are connected.

The relatively new field of energy medicine, which includes therapies like acupuncture, qigong, and therapeutic touch, aims to harness the universal energy that surrounds and penetrates the body to heal. One study, published in the journal *Evidence-Based Complementary and Alternative Medicine,* found that ten minutes of Reiki—a form of therapeutic touch in which energy is channeled through a healer's hands to a patient's body to promote healing—was as effective as physical therapy in improving the range of motion in people with mobility problems.

The Energy Body and Physical Health

Why does your energy body have such a profound influence on your flesh-and-bone body? Maybe because it was "born" first.

Your physical body came into being at the moment of your conception. But your energy body came first, formed by your biological parents' thoughts or feelings just before their egg and sperm united. An energy body "born" with wormholes—or one that acquires them after birth, via everyday stressors, may be the primary cause of physical symptoms or illnesses.

Your DNA contains all of the messages from your ancestors of all generations. It is unique to you—it has never been duplicated and never will be. Your DNA also has a distinct vibration, affected by your parents' conscious intentions.

The fields of psychoneuroimmunology and psychoendocrinology study the effects of the mind on the immune system and the endocrine system, respectively. The findings emerging from these disciplines are astonishing. For example, chronic depression increases the production of interleukin 6 (I-6), a chemical messenger for the immune system. Elevated IL-6 is associated with chronic inflammation, which, in turn, is implicated in many age-related diseases including heart disease, type 2 diabetes, arthritis, osteoporosis, and Alzheimer's disease, as we have seen.

In a study published in the journal *Psychoneuroendocrinology*, nineteen experienced practitioners of meditation practiced mindfulness meditation for one eight-hour day. A control group of twenty-one non-meditators did other leisure activities—they read, watched documentaries or played computer games, or walked. Afterward, everyone was asked to give a five-minute impromptu speech. Although meditation can't alter the fact that giving a speech without prep time is stressful, blood tests for the stress hormone cortisol showed that the meditators recovered from the stress more quickly than those in the control group.

It's my belief that the Apollo Factor can help DNA recall that unique "song" and change gene expression. That's what I believe the researchers in the study described above saw in the meditators—a reduction in the expression of several genes involved in regulating the inflammation and stress responses.

How You Feel Is How You Heal

As mentioned earlier, your mind—and therefore your thoughts, feelings, beliefs, intuition, and life experiences—"live" in your energy body. When you're in balance with your two bodies, your Apollo Factor is fully activated. Imbalances can affect your lifestyle choices, physiology, and health.

Your mind either affirms life or goes against it. For example, scientists at the the HeartMath Institute have found that positive emotions like love, gratitude, and joy raise levels of the hormone DHEA19 (which helps protect the body from stress) and an infection-fighting antibody called IgA, while negative emotions lower these substances.

Another study has linked positive emotions—especially the awe generated by the beauty of spirituality, nature, and art—with lower levels of pro-inflammatory cytokines (proteins that signal the immune system to work harder). In two experiments, more than two hundred adults reported the extent to which they'd experienced positive emotions that day. Then, samples of their gum and cheek tissue were taken. Those volunteers who'd reported experiencing the most positive feelings—including joy, love, contentment, and, particularly awe—had the lowest levels of the cytokine Interleukin 6, a marker of inflammation. I'd say that was the Apollo Factor at work!

Because your physical and energy bodies are connected, what happens to one affects the other. Steep your mind and energy body in love and joy, and you're going with energy of the universe. It gets us back to our cosmic song and DNA vibrating to its original perfect health and the organs and tissues of the body reverting back to a sense of well-being. When you retune your DNA to your cosmic song, source, and vibration, and tumors can experience apoptosis (programmed cell death), and health is restored.

But steeping the mind in negative thoughts and feelings—anger, anxiety, bitterness, or pain in your past—can lead to wormholes that damage the energetic "you" and weaken the Apollo Factor's healing potential. Had a migraine recently? Is your gastroesophageal reflux disease (GERD) acting up? Did your doctor just find a suspicious mole or lump? All originated as wormholes in your energy body, that Apollo Bridge. They took weeks, months, or years to show up in your physical body. And while the Apollo Factor doesn't normally improve or resolve symptoms or disease overnight, sometimes healing happens quicker than you'd think.

My Own Brush with Surgery

If I ever have my arm cut off, take me to the best surgeon around. But if I get sick, take me to my qigong master. Well, in 1998, Master Fu came to me—in the hospital.

I'd gone to the ER because I felt strange—clammy, a little weak, just not myself. The diagnosis: heart attack. I knew this wasn't true. Before I called 911, I'd given myself an electrocardiogram and tested levels of certain enzymes that, if high, would suggest injury to the heart. Both of these tests were normal. Still, the cardiologist recommended a cardiac catheterization.

"No," I said.

He persisted—without this procedure, he said, he could not guarantee my survival.

"No," I repeated. "This is not a heart attack."

My refusal was understandably frustrating for him. But because he believed that a patient has the right to participate in his own care, he agreed to abide by my wishes.

I was admitted to the intensive care unit for observation, and immediately raised eyebrows by asking Master Fu, my qigong teacher, to come in and evaluate me. He had taught me qigong exercises, and I had studied acupuncture under him. I wanted him to use Chinese pulse diagnosis to diagnose the problem. Would he agree with me that this was no heart attack but a far less serious condition?

Most of the nurses who had finished their shifts waited around for Master Fu to see what he would do. As I lay there hooked up to monitors, my teacher walked in, placed his hands over my body, and put his fingers on both my wrists to take the pulse—not to count my pulse rate, but to ascertain my levels of *qi* imbalance, and placed his hand on my chest.

"Your heart is fine," he said. "The problem is with your lungs—they have too much *qi*. Come see me when you leave the hospital."

Before I left, to satisfy my cardiologist, I had an electrocardiogram and a thallium stress test. Both were normal. He agreed to discharge me but stuck to his diagnosis that I'd had a "minor heart attack." I knew, though, that I'd had some sort of blockage of *qi* in my lungs. All my life, my lungs have been a "weak spot." I was diagnosed with asthma at the age of five, and though it improved in my teens, it had reappeared in my forties. I was under some significant emotional stress at that time, and I knew I'd be fine once my *qi* was flowing freely.

After my discharge, I started acupuncture treatments with Master Fu. Over the next six weeks, the *qi* began to flow, and I resumed my regular exercise routine.

A year later, as usual, I entered a competition that included a six-mile run, ninety minutes of kayaking, and a twelve-mile mountain-bike course. I did it again the following year. And at the age of seventy-eight, I'm still going strong. This is the Apollo Factor at work in my life.

Thus, to enjoy optimum health, our bodies must be in harmony, both with our surroundings, our connections to other people, and the universal energy that regulates all of these. Activating your Apollo Factor with the natural techniques here, working together, can facilitate this return to balance, improving your health and helping you prevent or treat disease, and live a long productive and happy life.

I hope to see you at 122.

—Robert D. Willix, Jr., MD
CEO/Founder of Enlightened Living Medicine
Chief Medical Officer of Hippocrates Health Institute
Chief Medical Officer of LiquIVida Lounge
April 2019

REFERENCES

INTRODUCTION

Tosato, M., et al. 2007. "The aging process and potential interventions to extend life expectancy." *Clinical Interventions in Aging* 2: 401–412.

CHAPTER 1
CAUSE 1: OXIDATION AND FREE RADICAL DAMAGE

Sun, N., et al. 2016. "The mitochondrial basis of aging." *Molecular Cell* 61: 654–666.

CHAPTER 2
SOLUTION: GEROPROTECTORS—THE NEXT GENERATION OF ANTIOXIDANTS

Allerton, T. D., et al. 2018. "L-citrulline supplementation: impact on cardiometabolic health." *Nutrients* 10: 1–24.

Moss, J. W. E., et al. 2018. "Nutraceuticals as therapeutic agents for atherosclerosis." *BBA—Molecular Basis of Disease* 1864: 1562–1572.

Hernández-Camacho, J. D., et al. 2018. "Coenzyme Q10 supplementation in aging and disease." *Frontiers in Physiology* 9: 44.

Sadowska-Bartosz, I., and Bartosz, G. 2014. "Effect of antioxidants supplementation on aging and longevity." *BioMed Research International* 2014: 1–17.

Sia, H., and Liub, D. 2014. "Dietary anti-aging phytochemicals and mechanisms associated with prolonged survival." *Journal of Nutritional Biochemistry* 25: 581–591.

CHAPTER 3
CAUSE 2: **INFLAMMATION**

Balistreri, C. R. 2018. "Anti-inflamm-ageing and/or anti-age-related disease emerging treatments: a historical alchemy or revolutionary effective procedures?" *Mediators of Inflammation* 2018: 1–13.

Carey, N. *The Epigenetics Revolution*. New York: Columbia University Press, 2012.

Eger, H., et al. 2004. "The influence of being physically near to a cell phone transmission mast on the incidence of cancer." *Umwelt·Medizin·Gesellschaft* 17: 1–17.

Visser, M. 1999. "Elevated C-reactive protein levels in overweight and obese adults." *Journal of the American Medical Society* 282: 2131–2135.

Xia, S., et al. 2016. "An update on inflamm-aging: mechanisms, prevention, and treatment." *Journal of Immunology Research* 2016: 1–12.

CHAPTER 4
SOLUTION: **INFLAMMABOTS—THE NEW INFLAMMATION FIGHTERS**

Estruch, R., et al. 2018. "Primary prevention of cardiovascular disease with a Mediterranean diet supplemented with extra-virgin olive oil or nuts." *New England Journal of Medicine* 378: 1–25.

Ghanim, H., et al. 2009. "Increase in plasma endotoxin concentrations and the expression of Toll-like receptors and suppressor of cytokine signaling-3 in mononuclear cells after a high-fat, high-carbohydrate meal: implications for insulin resistance." *Diabetes Care* 32: 2281–2287.

CHAPTER 5
CAUSE 3: **DECLINING HORMONES AND PEPTIDES**

Amitani, M. et al. 2017. "The role of ghrelin and ghrelin signaling in aging." *International Journal of Molecular Sciences* 18: 1–18.

Banks, W. A., et al. 2010. "Effects of a growth hormone-releasing hormone antagonist on telomerase activity, oxidative stress, longevity, and aging in mice."

Proceedings of the National Academy of Science 107: 22272–22277.

Files, J. A. 2011. "Bioidentical hormone therapy; concise review for clinicians." *Mayo Clinic Proceedings* 86: 673–680.

Kumar, M., et al. 2016. "Human gut microbiota and healthy aging: recent developments and future prospective." *Nutrition and Healthy Aging* 4: 3–16.

Medeiros, A., and Watkins, E. S. 2018. "Live longer better: the historical roots of human growth hormone as anti-aging." *Medicine Journal of the History of Medicine and Allied Sciences* 73: 333–359.

Predrag, S., et al. 2016. "Brain-gut axis and pentadecapeptide BPC 157: theoretical and practical implications." *Current Neuropharmacology* 14: 857–865.

Reiter, R.J., et al. 2018. "Mitochondria: central organelles for melatonin's antioxidant and anti-aging actions." *Molecules* 23: 1–25.

Sigalos, J. T., et al. 2017. "Growth hormone secretagogue treatment in hypogonadal men raises serum insulin-like growth gactor-1 levels." *American Journal of Men's Health* 11: 1752–1757.

CHAPTER 6
SOLUTION: **STRENGTHEN THE HORMONE-PEPTIDE CONNECTION**

Kreatsoulas, C. and Anand, S. S. 2013. "Menopausal hormone therapy for the primary prevention of chronic conditions"; U.S. Preventive Services Task Force Recommendation Statement. *Polskie Archiwum Medycyny Wewnetrznej* 123: 112–116.

Moskowitz. D. 2006. "A comprehensive review of the safety and efficacy of bioidentical hormones for the management of menopause and related health risk." *Alternative Medicine Review* 11: 208–223.

Rudman, D. 1990. "Effects of Human Growth Hormone in Men over 60 Years Old." *The New England Journal of Medicine* 323: 1–6.

Samaras, N., et al. 2014. "Off-label use of hormones as an anti-aging strategy: a review." *Clinical Interventions in Aging* 9: 1175–1186.

CHAPTER 7

CAUSE 4: **SHORTENED TELOMERES**

Gomez, D. E. 2012. "Telomere structure and telomerase in health and disease (review)." *International Journal of Oncology* 41: 1561–1569.

Shay, J. W. 2016. "Role of telomeres and telomerase in aging and cancer." *Cancer Discovery* 6: 584–593.

Willeit, P., et al. 2010. "Telomere length and risk of incident cancer and cancer mortality. *Journal of the American Medical Association* 304: 69–75.

CHAPTER 8
SOLUTION: **TELOMERASE ACTIVATORS**

Balan, E., et al. 2018. "Physical activity and nutrition: two promising strategies for telomere maintenance." *Nutrients* 10: 1–14.

Challem, J. 2018. "The telomere treatment." *www.amazingwellnessmag.com.*

Conklin, Q/A., et al. 2018. "Insight meditation and telomere biology: The effects of intensive retreat and the moderating role of personality." *Brain, Behavior, and Immunity* 70: 233–245.

Emanuele, E., et al. 2013. "Topical application of preparations containing DNA repair enzymes prevents ultraviolet-induced telomere shortening and c-FOS proto-oncogene hyperexpression in human skin: an experimental pilot study." *Journal of Drugs in Dermatology* 12: 1017–1021.

Jaskelioff, M., et al. 2011. "Telomerase reactivation reverses tissue degeneration in aged telomerase-deficient mice." *Nature* 469: 102–106.

Leung, C. W., et al. 2014. "Soda and cell aging: association between sugar-sweetened beverage consumption and leukocyte telomere length in healthy adults from the National Health and Nutrition Examination Surveys." *American Journal of Public Health* 104: 2425–2431.

Lohner, S., et al. 2017. "Health outcomes of non-nutritive sweeteners: analysis of the research landscape." *Nutrition Journal* 16: 55.

O'Callaghan, N., et al. 2014. "Telomere shortening in elderly individuals with mild cognitive impairment may be attenuated with ω-3 fatty acid supplementation: a randomized controlled pilot study." *Nutrition* 30: 489–491.

Salvador, L., et al. 2016. "A natural product telomerase activator lengthens telomeres in humans: a randomized, double blind, and placebo controlled study." *Rejuvenation Research* 19: 478–484.

Sjogren, P., et al. 2014. "Stand up for health—avoiding sedentary behaviour might lengthen your telomeres: secondary outcomes from a physical activity RCT in older people." *British Journal of Sports Medicine* 48: 1407–1409.

Verhoeven, J. E., et al. 2014. "Major depressive disorder and accelerated cellular aging: results from a large psychiatric cohort study." *Molecular Psychiatry* 19(8): 895–901.

Zhu, H., et al. 2011. "Increased telomerase activity and vitamin D supplementation in overweight African Americans." *International Journal of Obesity* 36: 805–809.

CHAPTER 9
CAUSE 5: **PHYSICAL INACTIVITY**

Keadle, S. K., et al. 2015. "Impact of changes in television viewing time and physical activity on longevity: a prospective cohort study." *International Journal of Behavioral Nutrition and Physical Activity* 12: 156.

CHAPTER 10
SOLUTION: **ANTI-AGING EXERCISE**

Garatachea, N., et al. 2015. "Exercise attenuates the major hallmarks of aging." *Rejuvenation Research* 18: 57–89.

Gass, R. 2004. "Tai Chi Chuan and bone loss in postmenopausal women." *Archives of Physical Medicine and Rehabilitation* 84: 621.

Tolahunase, M, et al. 2017. "Impact of yoga and meditation on cellular aging in apparently healthy individuals: a prospective, open-label single-arm exploratory study." *Oxidative Medicine and Cellular Longevity*, Epub January 16.

CHAPTER 11
CAUSE 6: **SEVEN NUTRITIONAL PITFALLS THAT PROMOTE AGING**

Martins, M., et al. 2017. "A new approach to assess lifetime dietary patterns finds lower consumption of animal foods with aging in a longitudinal analysis of a health-oriented Adventist population." *Nutrients* 9: 1118 1–16.

Nettleton, J. A., et al. 2008. "Dietary patterns, food groups, and telomere length in the Multi-Ethnic Study of Atherosclerosis (MESA)." *American Journal of Clinical Nutrition* 88: 1405–1412.

Nicholls, S. J., et al. 2006. "Consumption of saturated fat impairs the anti-inflammatory properties of high-density lipoproteins and endothelial function." *Journal of the American College of Cardiology* 48: 715–20.

Satija, A., and Hu, F. B. 2018. "Plant-based diets and cardiovascular health." *Trends in Cardiovascular Medicine* 28: 437–441.

CHAPTER 12
SOLUTION: **REJUVENATION NUTRITION**

Cederholm, T., and Morley, J. E. 2016. "Nutrient interface with biology and aging." *Current Opinion in Clinical Nutrition and Metabolic Care* 19: 1–4.

Craig, D., et al. 2014. "Healthy aging diets other than the Mediterranean: a focus on the Okinawan diet." *Mechanisms of Ageing and Development*, March/April: 136–137: 148–162.

Manach, C., et al. 2017. "Addressing the inter-individual variation in response to consumption of plant food bioactives: towards a better understanding of their role in healthy aging and cardiometabolic risk reduction." *Molecular Nutrition & Food Research* 61: 1–16, Epub November 15.

Masoro, E. J. 2003. "Subfield history: caloric restriction, slowing aging, and extending life." *Science of Aging Knowledge Environment*, February 26: RE2.

Seidelmann, S.B., et al. 2018. "Dietary carbohydrate intake and mortality: a prospective cohort study and meta-analysis." *Lancet Public Health* 3: e419-e428.

CHAPTER 13
CAUSE 7: **STRESS**

Rahe, R. H., and Arthur, R. J. 1978. "Life change and illness studies: Past history and future directions." *Journal of Human Stress* 4: 3–15.

Tobias, E., et al. 2018. "Chromosomal processes in mind-body medicine: chronic stress, cell aging, and telomere length." *Medical Science Monitor Basic Review* 24: 134–140.

CHAPTER 14
SOLUTION: AGE-DEFYING STRESS MANAGEMENT

Rao, R. V. 2018. "Ayurveda and the science of aging." *Journal of Ayurveda and Integrative Medicine* 9: 225–232.

CHAPTER 16
THE APOLLO FACTOR: RECLAIMING YOUR COSMIC GIFT OF SELF-HEALING

Aanwar, Y. 2015. "Add nature, art and religion to life's best anti-inflammatories." *Berkeley News*, February 2.

Chittaranjan Andrade, C. and Radhakrishnan, R. 2009. "Prayer and healing: A medical and scientific perspective on randomized controlled trials." *Indian Journal of Psychiatry* 51: 247–253.

Elkins, G., et al. 2009. "Hypnotherapy for the Management of Chronic Pain." *The International Journal of Clinical and Experimental Hypnosis* 55: 275–287.

Herreros-Villanueva, M., et al. 2012. "Spontaneous regression of pancreatic cancer: real or a misdiagnosis?" *World Journal of Gastroenterology* 18: 2902–2908.

Sloan, R. P., and Ramakrishnan, R. 2012. "Science, medicine, and intercessory prayer." *Perspectives in Biology and Medicine* 49: 504–514.

Turan, B., et al. 2015. "Anticipatory sensitization to repeated stressors: the role of initial cortisol reactivity and meditation/emotion skills training." *Psychoneuroendocrinology* 52: 229–238.

ABOUT THE AUTHOR

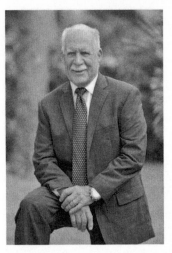

Robert D. Willix, Jr, MD, formerly a Board Certified cardiac surgeon, pioneered the first open heart surgery program in South Dakota. After developing the Cardiac Rehabilitation Human Performance Program at the North Broward Hospital District during the 1980s, he turned his focus to prevention.

With a passion for integrative healing, Dr. Willix traveled the world to study acupuncture, Ayurvedic Medicine, and the healing ways of Shamanism from the Inka tradition. He is currently one of 300 physicians in the United States who is trained in Pulse Diagnosis and he learned a specialized form of acupuncture from world-famous qigong Master, Master Fu.

He is CEO of Enlightened Living Medicine and the Chief Medical Officer and Director of Energy Medicine at the world-famous Hippocrates Health Institute in Palm Beach, Florida. He is also CMO of LiquIVida Lounge, a company devoted to teaching people that they control their own health destiny. He is an avid athlete, having completed fourteen marathons and the Ironman Triathlon in Kona, Hawaii.

ACKNOWLEDGMENTS

It has been said that "It takes a village to raise a child."

"It takes several villages: patience, brutal honesty, fortitude, luck, and love to raise an author to write a book."

—Robert D. Willix, Jr., MD

I want to share this project with all the villagers in my tribe.

My wife, France Toupin Willix, put her life on hold to support this book from beginning to end. For her painstaking attention to detail and the courage to put up with me for this last year plus.

To Maggie Greenwood-Robinson, whose literary knowledge, unwavering belief, and ability helped me when I would lose my vision. She is one of the only reasons this project was completed. I believe that she has not only made me a better author, but has me hoping our work together has just begun. Thank you, Maggie, for your tireless assistance, friendship, laughter, and dedication to *The Rejuvenation Solution*.

Thank you to all the staff at HCI Books, the copy editors for their ability to see beyond spell check and correcting the order of the written word. The art direction of Larissa at HCI was appreciated very much. She has accepted my inability to draw and yet make the book's illustrations so perfect.

A very special thank you for the editorial direction of Allison Janse. She accepted my manuscript from the very first time she read it and has guided us all through the deadlines with her patience and caring manner. The cover design is a direct tribute to her persistence—thank you!

Last but not least, is the direction and fortitude of my agent Steve Troha. He never gave up over the last several years, getting this work to as many publishers as would take a chance. I can only believe that this is just the beginning of a long friendship.

Please forgive me if I have accidentally left someone out because this truly has been a journey not an event.

Thank you, all!!

Dr. Bob Willix

INDEX

247